Please Read This Leaflet Carefully

Karen Havelin

dead ink

dead ink

Copyright © Karen Havelin 2019
All rights reserved.

This is a work of fiction.

The right of Karen Havelin to be identified as the author of this work has been asserted by her in accordance with the Copyright, Designs and Patents Act 1988.

First published in Great Britain in 2019 by Dead Ink, an imprint of Cinder House Publishing Limited.

ISBN 9781911585541

Cover design by Luke Bird
lukebird.co.uk

Printed and bound in Great Britain by Clays Ltd, Elcograf S.p.A

www.deadinkbooks.com

What you say, you say in a body; you can say nothing outside of this body.

—Plate 59, plate 105
The Gospel of Philip

You do not have to be good.
You do not have to walk on your knees
for a hundred miles through the desert repenting.
You only have to let the soft animal of your body
love what it loves.

—Mary Oliver

PART I

NOW MY HEART IS FULL

2016

For years, I've considered it an established fact that the female body is a pain in the ass. Despite all its unique talents, from youth it's constantly wracked by hurricanes, snow and rain—by cramps and pains, premenstrual craziness, menstrual craziness, postmenstrual craziness, pill-related craziness; waves of uncontrollable rage and sadness, fluctuating weight and libido, urinary tract infections, yeast infections, not to mention the smorgasbord of mindboggling changes that is pregnancy. There are so many things that swell, ache, cramp and droop. So many places an eponymous cancer can settle—breasts, uterus, ovaries—and so many illnesses that are specifically female. The male body seems like a sunny campsite in comparison.

My feet are in the cold, metal stirrups.

"Has it been a whole year? That must be a good sign, huh?"

"Yeah, I've been doing okay."

My gynecologist signals me towards her with an efficient, little wave of her fingers and I scoot further down on the table.

Beneath me, the paper cover crunches against the padded vinyl seat. My doctor is an intelligent woman with a slight accent, who never appears to be in a hurry. She is in her early sixties and has a smooth, gray bob and a pleasant face untouched by Botox. I think she's had a happy life.

I lean back and focus on the irregularly sized holes in the ceiling tiles, trying not to tense up against the business end of the speculum. Luckily, she knows what she's doing and it barely hurts.

"How's the little one?"

"She's great. She's two already."

"Still not decided on having more?"

Her voice is coming from down between my ankles.

"Uh, I just got divorced actually, so I have enough on my plate right now."

Telling people about my divorce while my bodily cavities are propped open feels like one step too far.

"Oh. Well, you're only thirty-five, you have time."

Fortunately, my doctor is quick. She finishes taking the sample and finally removes the speculum. She lowers the lights and prepares the ultrasound wand by squirting gel on it.

"So, are we losing you to Norway?"

"No, no danger of that yet."

I've only gone back once after I left at twenty-nine, six years ago. My family has consistently lobbied me to move back home ever since I got my master's degree. They doubled down on their pleas when Nick and I split up and I became alone with Ella most of the time.

As she begins the ultrasound examination, I watch the shapes of my inner organs balloon like elusive deep-sea creatures against the murky display. I chew my lip and think I see something unfamiliar, but then again, I always do. It's beyond me how she can make any sense of these images.

"How's it looking?"

She's quiet for a while, clicking and dragging the measurement line against one shape.

"Hmm, it looks like there's a small cyst. But it should disappear on its own."

"So, it's not like the previous ones."

"No."

"Does that mean I shouldn't worry?"

"Yes. How is your pain these days?"

"Good, by my standards. I keep up the meditation, acupuncture, that sort of thing. But it's been better since the pregnancy. I'm just worried that it won't last."

Actually, I haven't seen my acupuncturist in a long time, which is maybe a sign of improved health in itself.

"Still, you seem to be doing surprisingly well," the doctor says as I sit up, fussing with the hospital gown so that it spreads down to my knees.

"Try not to worry. You never worry about the right things anyway, my mother always said."

Well.

Still, I leave her office feeling basically intact as I walk a few avenues west to catch the subway home. I am glad to be in New York, despite how exhausting it sometimes is to maintain life here. As long as I can keep my health insurance, there's undeniable glamour in having these giant, iconic buildings and straight, gingko tree-lined streets be the set for our daily life. I notice the late afternoon sunlight reflecting off the buildings as I cross an avenue; and as the yellow cabs swarm at the stoplight, I get that sense of spaciousness, of being the main character in a movie, and reflect that fourteen-year-old me would have loved this. She was obsessed with things being beautiful and exciting, always eager to be delighted. How hopeful that girl was. The chain of things I wanted when I was younger, the links stretching backwards to angrier, more innocent and optimistic versions of me.

Back on the Upper West Side, my upstairs neighbors are watching Ella. They've fed her dinner and she's ready for bed. When Madeline opens the door to let me in, Ella is sitting on her backpack in the hallway of their apartment. The hallway is dark and cramped, the floor covered in shoes of all sizes. I hear Madeline's husband laugh in the other room and the chirps of their youngest, Sophie. My heart lifts and simultaneously aches at the sight of Ella's tiny legs in her little jeans. She turns her round, blue eyes to me and runs over and hugs my legs, pressing her face against my thighs. I put a hand on her warm, silky head.

"She's insisted on waiting for you in the hallway since dinner," Madeline says with a resigned smile. That's my girl. So shy but so firm. I squat down to kiss her hair and poke her belly gently. To avoid allergic reactions, I usually try to embrace her without touching my bare skin to her before I can change her clothes and give her a bath. But she gives me a secret, bright smile and I lift her, squeezing her warm, little body against mine, feeling her hands and her face against my neck. I thank Madeline before we head downstairs to our apartment, Ella's backpack, coat and boots clasped in my other hand.

"Did you have fun, *lillepus*?" I ask her in the stairwell.

She shakes her head.

"Not even a little bit? Not even with the cat?"

"The cat's name is Joe!"

I fiddle with the lock and, in the end, I have to put her down. I breathe a sigh of relief as I close the door behind us and take in the familiar smells of our tiny apartment: clean laundry, yesterday's cooking, and the warm, sweet scent of her.

I take off my coat and get a wet wipe to wash her face and hands. I know I'll have painful, itchy patches of bright red allergic reactions on the skin of my neck all night because of hugging her earlier, even though I am washing my skin now. Children are of the moment. Either you're there with them or you're not.

Death drop: Similar to the back sit-spin; it involves a jump, as in the flying camel, but the skater drops immediately to a back sit position.

— Skate:100 Years of Figure Skating by Steve Milton

I try to talk to my sister Ingrid as well as one of my parents each weekend. They divorced many years ago, a decision that was probably wise, but handled badly. I run all medical news past my father, who's a doctor. He must worry, but he never tells me, for which I'm grateful. My conversations with my mother, who's a nurse, usually revolve around other people we know. On Sunday morning, I sit on the sofa in the living room in front of my laptop. It's a bright day and there are plush toys strewn around. I can see the wooden panels on the wall behind my mother on the screen. She is planning her retirement in a few years. It's a rainy day in Bergen and she has begun to pick the invasive Iberia slugs from her garden for the season.

Her voice goes up an octave when she talks to Ella. She always speaks Norwegian, though Ella replies in English. I try to let them talk amongst themselves, but they both seem to want me in the mix. Ella finishes telling her about our neighbor's cat before suddenly feeling shy and wandering off. I ask about my aunt Elsa. I rearrange my hair so it won't look so flat in the little window of myself on the screen and try to think of something to say to end the call. Instead, my mother takes charge.

"So, how are you?"

"I'm okay. Just exhausted."

"Well, if you lived closer, I could help you out more." Her voice is tense. I don't have a lot of adult conversations with my mother, because once Ella goes to bed, when it would be natural to have those conversations, my mother is fast asleep, six hours ahead of us in Norway. I feel the weight of being the only parent in the room these days, always responsible, but remembering my mother talking about how much she sacrificed for me doesn't help. It only makes it clearer that, most of the time, there is no way of getting across the gulfs between people.

"Maybe I could take a little trip next month and help you out a bit," she suggests, but then pauses. "Or, well, that's close to the summer. I'll have to look at tickets."

I wish she could be here tomorrow and just take control of everything the way she did when Ella was a newborn. The sudden longing makes me want to cry.

"That would be nice."

My voice cracks embarrassingly, which we both ignore.

She studies my face carefully on the screen.

"Oh, by the way!"

My mother pixelates a little and her voice in the speakers turns clangy so I don't catch what she's saying at first—only the name Kjetil.

"What, *my* Kjetil?"

"Yeah, he's moving to New York for work."

I don't know what to say. I don't even know what Kjetil does these days, but six years ago it was completely and thoroughly impossible for him to find a job in New York.

"Uh. That's nice for him."

"He's divorced, you know. He wanted a change is what Janne said. Wanted to get out of Norway. Well, *you* get it."

"Yeah."

I note the intensity of my emotions, the familiar mix of bitterness and sadness tempered with what my life is now—Ella, New York City, responsibilities, adulthood. Something like fear. But there's a little sliver of panicky excitement too.

All day, I try unsuccessfully to put Kjetil out of my mind.

I wake up Monday morning, after a night of chaotic dreams, and my shoulders and arms, which have been painful for weeks, feel even worse. My right shoulder and my lower arms are cold, stiff countries of their own. Other days, they feel hot and nauseating. How am I going to get through the work week like this? I look up a local clinic to start the physical therapy I've been putting off for weeks. Luckily, they have an opening for tomorrow afternoon.

Ella is two. She is very pale and often shy around other people. Nick worries that she's too quiet, but I don't think so. It's a cultural difference, too. In Norway, being quiet is always the lesser crime. She seems sharper than other kids her age, at least to me. She just likes to think things through on her own before talking. She looks like me at that age. Her hair is fine and light and her eyes a clear blue. In winter, she sometimes reminds me of a little jellyfish. She's exquisitely formed, neither plump nor limp, but her small features appear to be made of something a tiny bit too frail. As though, if you pricked her, clear liquid would leak out and she would disappear completely. When I see her picking at her oatmeal in the mornings, I always think of what my mother used to say to me when I was an underweight child who hated eating:

"You have to eat your dinner or you'll shrink until there's nothing left of you but a little wet spot!"

Mornings alone with Ella are my favorite time of day. I pad quietly into her bedroom, a tiny alcove with yellow wallpaper. The apartment was too small for us before Nick moved out. I lift Ella out of her bed in the corner and carry the sleep-scented bundle of her into the warm bathroom, then set her carefully down on her feet in the middle of the floor. Ella stands there quietly blinking and yawning while I unbutton her footie pajamas and dress her. NPR plays at low volume on the radio. It takes about half an hour before Ella starts speaking in the mornings. Before that, the only noise that comes from her is the sound of her small breaths when my ear is next to her mouth. She is perfectly self-contained, a peaceful little animal.

Now My Heart Is Full

On Tuesday, when it's time for physical therapy, I leave work early to locate the building on the Upper West side. In the small waiting room that still has Christmas lights up, I notice I'm the only person under fifty. Uncomfortable chairs with wooden armrests line the walls. As usual, I'm too short to reach the floor and the back of the chair at the same time. I perch on the front of the seat, with my legs crossed. The low table in the center of the room is covered in interior design magazines for people who own property. No one in this room does, I feel fairly certain, but I tensely flip through one as I wait. I scan photos of all the different landscapes people wake up to— properties in Dallas, Naples, Switzerland—vast foyers and wide, sweeping staircases, empty white walls, high ceilings, shiny parquet floors, sunlight spilling in from green gardens. Imagine filling those large spaces with your personality.

I haven't seen a new medical professional on my own in a while and even when it was a common occurrence in my late twenties and early thirties, I never stopped being nervous. It felt like I was waiting for an exam, a moment to perform and be judged. Since Ella's birth, life has been miraculously uneventful when it comes to my health. I read somewhere that stress can worsen endometriosis, even bring forth cysts— now there's a thought that brings a surge of cortisol. I try to stop this line of thinking there, but of course I can't. The echo of hospital corridors, bright overhead lights, texture of institutional sheets, and that nauseous 4 a.m. feeling crowd in on me. I look at the other people in the waiting room, the middle-aged man with the cane and the tiny, hunched old woman, imagining the suffering that brings them here. What do we do when health runs out?

Finally, a young woman comes out and calls out: "Laura Fuh-juh…?"

I correct her automatically: "Fjellstad, yes. Like in 'fjord.' It's Norwegian."

I saw a physical therapist ten years ago in Norway, but she was a different breed than this polished, pony-tailed professional, who introduces herself as Chelsea and leads me into a shabby room with a low ceiling filled with benches and exercise equipment. The room feels dim, even under the wash of fluorescence. When I look at the objects in the room, I can't identify what exactly makes it all feel so scruffy. Nothing is in and of itself shabby. The floor that, at first glance, looks like old cracked linoleum is in fact made up of thick, shock-absorbing rubber squares that fit together like puzzle pieces, and the benches and the machines aren't too worn, either. There's a pile of white towels on a table. A large man with an even larger shirt and droopy shoulders is folding another pile of white towels, making a rough stack.

Chelsea sits me down on a plastic chair and picks up a clipboard. She has broad cheekbones, expertly applied eye shadow, and long ash blonde hair tied in a swinging ponytail. She speaks quickly, smiling with slightly crooked teeth, every sentence ending on an up.

"So, what have we here?" she says.

"Well, I've been having pain in my shoulders and arms for a while." I touch my shoulders awkwardly. "But lately it's making it hard to work, so…tendonitis apparently."

"What kind of work do you do?"

"I do administrative office work—it's all on the computer."

In fact, despite my efforts, ever since my pregnancy, my posture has become molded forward more and more, into an increasingly defeated hunch with a touch of gorilla. I'm by no means fat, but my shape feels slightly wrong; clothes don't suit me as well as they used to.

"This is what we call a defensive posture?" Chelsea says. "Your shoulders coming forward make your chin come forward too, which shortens the muscles in the back of your neck?"

She tests my arms by squeezing them different ways, telling me to resist the pressure and to let her know if anything is painful. As she bends over me, I can't help but notice how lovely the skin on Chelsea's neck is, smooth and slightly pearlescent. I certainly don't begrudge anyone their youthfully slim plumpness; their wealth of collagen. She has an inkling that my real problem isn't where it hurts the most. She traces the pain from my tingling fingers; it travels straight up my wrists and winds itself tightly around my upper arms diagonally like ribbons on a ballet slipper. The ribbons circle my shoulders and continue down my back to between the shoulder blades. There, they form a grid of tension around the spine where it pools before the concave of the neck. Higher up, the grid turns into a tight brace around the neck, the muscles where my body becomes my head are hard and numb.

My eyes follow Chelsea as she starts to take notes on her clipboard.

"Is there any hope for me?" I smile faintly.

Chelsea gives me a friendly smile that's only a tiny bit patronizing.

"If you do your exercises and ice your shoulders a lot, we'll fix you right up!"

She attaches wires to my neck, covers them with heat packs she picks out of a steaming vat, and wraps me in towels.

She starts up the electric stimulation massage and increases its power click by click until my neck starts buzzing. It's a strange sensation, but not unpleasant. The warmth, gentle buzzing, and soothing weight of the pack makes my eyelids sink. Sitting still on the chair amidst bantering employees and patients—being where I'm supposed to be without having to do anything—is wonderful.

Chelsea hops up on the bench behind my chair for the five-minute massage that comes after. Her hands are strong, and within seconds find a frozen knot between my shoulder and neck. She chats to her colleague about her gel manicure. All I can do is sit still and close my eyes, desperate for the massage to continue, even though it's painful.

It's darker than normal behind my eyelids, and suddenly he's there: Kjetil. The comforting pull of him, his warmth, the scent of his skin, his voice and laugh. But there is the terrible soreness of it too, like the taste of blood. When I moved here without Kjetil, it wasn't just getting over one relationship and going on to the next. It's as if I drowned crossing the Atlantic Ocean and this is an entirely different life.

When the massage ends, I open my eyes and feel disoriented, like I've been asleep.

Chelsea tells me to sit at the arm bike, which is exactly what the name suggests. I feel silly making big circles with my arms to move the pedals, like I'm cartoon-swimming.

"Do you work out?" Chelsea asks.

"Well, I try, but it's not so easy for a single mother," I say in a voice that sounds strange even to me. I feel tenderized, weird, on the verge of tears. I know this twenty-five-year-old won't have anything to offer by way of comfort. Still, I find I want something from her—from her bright, uncomplicated world where nothing is broken.

"Aw, well," Chelsea says, unmoved. "Let me see if I can't come up with some exercises you can do at home!"

I resume biking, feeling chastened.

The arm problem seems to be divorce-related: it reappeared for the first time in years around the same time Nick and I split up. My posture deteriorated along with the relationship. I've tried to keep it under control with an occasional massage and some vaguely remembered exercises, but for weeks now, my arms have been painful even at the beginning of the workday.

My marriage let me pretend to be a normal person for a few years. There was the happy start; of gulping down everything simple and tasty after being heartbroken over Kjetil and years of illness. Then, getting pregnant without having to go through IVF was such a stroke of magical luck that I let go of how much easier it all would've been if I'd been in my home country. I was able to lay any doubts about my location in the world and the father of my child completely to rest. It felt like the exercises I learned to do to avoid eye strain while working on the computer: turn away from the screen and let my eyes land on something far away. My eye muscles would strain to see rooftops in the distance before suddenly, blissfully, remember how to relax on the blue, clear sky. That feeling of more territory, regained space—I'd remember how to straighten my spine and take a deep breath, how to live in the world.

I could make peace with anything as long as I could have Ella.

In time, though, there was only a lack of resonance and a constant supply of irritation between Nick and me. It was not true love. It was something smaller.

"Some people can't handle child-rearing," my mother had said, in that way that is meant to be supportive but comes with the aftertaste of criticism.

"You know statistically that's when people go nuts, right?"

In my mind, the failure of our marriage hinged on him giving in to the temptation of secretly believing my illness was my fault. That there was some abstract, heroic, grand gesture to be performed, but I refused to do it. He would resist the drudgery of the ongoing pain by thinking that if the roles were reversed, he would have solved it all, somehow. To be fair, Nick probably didn't really realize what being ill meant until after Ella was born and we were so overwhelmed that neither of us could hide unappealing traits for long.

Just as well to be alone.

I'm lucky that he is neither unstable nor gratuitously mean. At times, I dare to think that the worst of it is over. I've stopped running my tongue over the wound. The way we share Ella seems more or less right. We both watch her closely but she seems to be doing okay so far. I work full time at Scandinavia House—but Nick works long hours and travels a lot, so Ella is still mine most of the time.

Once I got my new life stumbling along on its newborn calf legs, it was a relief to live alone again—not the gaping hole of loneliness, with double the difficulties, that I'd feared. In between the heartbreak and the dark thoughts that still dominate, there are pauses. I've picked up writing again. After I make it through the mornings, the commute, and workday, getting us both home and fed and Ella to sleep, there is occasionally a tiny space in which I am alone with myself. I'm exhausted, but every once in a while, I wipe the kitchen table and sit down for a half an hour and put my hands on the keyboard of my aging laptop. I leave old manuscripts alone and just type. After a while, something flows through me, like I've plugged into a current. It's a profound relief to not be disturbed. Old creative muscles reawaken and it's downright joyful to see that I can still write—even after two years where it seemed like I gave up everything I had to have my daughter. There is privacy in my own head—I wait and see if anything will happen; I trust the process of it. I don't have to show it to anyone, but it's not nothing—at times it's just a random flow of descriptive or exclaiming words, and at times it's something tiny and green that unfurls slowly. Other times it's something dark and large that makes a racket falling down the stairs, threatening to break things in its path. Whatever I create is only mine.

Over the next few days, I feel vaguely out of control. There are stretches of unbidden daydreams of my early days with Kjetil, when we were still students. He was so happy and generous. Waking up in his room with sunlight pouring in, turning over to see his smiling, brown eyes right there, his hands and his warm hairiness, how our bodies fit together so well, so much kissing that the scratchiness of his chin gave me a rash. He would grow stubbly by the evening even with a daily morning shave, so he approached his shaving ritual with precision—that neat line of black hair at his temples and neck, even when he was a student and everyone else in Bergen was wearing their hair seventies-style shaggy. I remember the sensation of his smooth skin against my lips as I kissed the back of his neck. It's s so vivid even after all these years that it feels dangerous. I've worked very hard to close that part of the past off and managing to do so was a question of survival. It's so delicious to crack the door a little. All the color and light that comes from there.

One evening, I almost fall asleep when I put Ella to bed, but instead I get up and call my friend Tatiana to talk to an adult. I tell her a little of the story of Kjetil while cleaning up the kitchen and she asks why I don't just call him up. I sit down on the sofa. My living room is a mess, still too empty in places yet cluttered with toys, magazines, and clothes. I lean my head against the wall behind the sofa and stare at the patchy ceiling.

"Because it almost killed me when it ended," I say, aware that I sound melodramatic.

Do I want to talk to him? No. Too risky. I should ask my mother what neighborhood he lives in. I could probably avoid ever seeing him if I didn't contact him. Kjetil met his wife right after I left the country. There was some overlap of these relationships after I had left, but before we broke up officially. It was a period in our lives when neither of us handled anything particularly well. Still, I have considerable bitterness about these things. It feels cold and stuck, and sometimes hot and nauseous, like my right shoulder. Tatiana knows I had surgeries for endometriosis before I came to the US and that chronic pain was more of an issue when I first arrived than it is now. She knows that I still have to ration my energy and be careful about everything and still, regardless of what I do, pain still claims a certain percentage of my life. But even when someone knows the details of my illness, even if they were interested in understanding it—a tiny group of people—how could I make them understand what sort of world I was living in at the time? I could barely rest because the pain was constant. I felt like I couldn't breathe, like there wasn't enough light in the world.

"I was sick," I say to Tatiana. "I never thought I'd have even this much of a normal life."

Tatiana is silent.

"I don't even know if he'd want to talk to me. He was so angry too, when I ended it."

"Well, you're not going to know unless you try, right?" Tatiana says, eager to end this conversation with a positive spin. "Have you given any more thought to getting a dating profile like I told you to? Maybe it would take your mind off things. Or motivate you to call him. Being single in your thirties is not the same as in your twenties, believe me."

The thought of trying to make myself attractive to strangers is daunting, to say the least. The private palenesses, smells, and tender spots of other people's bodies. The last time I actively dated was before I met Kjetil. How bright and easy my life was back then—how miraculously comfortable I was with him. During the first orgasm he ever gave me, in his dark bedroom with the lights of passing cars flickering across the ceiling, I kept seeing myself on the ice rink, trying and trying to get a difficult pirouette right, almost getting it but losing speed, almost, *almost*—then by waiting a millisecond longer to switch legs and using my arms to harness all that speed, *finally*—perfect, glorious spinning, balanced as if it could go on forever. That was just the beginning. The mere presence of his body seemed to put mine at ease.

I'd fled all my ties in Norway, but when I became a mother, I found taking care of a vulnerable baby surprisingly doable. People say no one talks about the worst parts of childcare, but it seemed like I hardly heard anything else before having a kid. People who expect the pregnant body to be graceful and wise, who go in expecting parenting to run smoothly and to always be flooded by feelings of joy and rightness, have had a different kind of life than mine. I spent the thirty hours of her birth in a state of suspended dread, receiving help from the nice nurses at every turn, just like I had during my surgeries, and was happy that we both came out of it alive and me with about the same amount of hospital-related PTSD as before.

After years of thinking that needing help or caring for other people would be the worst thing in the world, Ella's arrival in my life was something of a revelation. Taking care of her was not impossible. I did not resent her for needing me. Being needed every second of the day felt confining, exhausting and overwhelming at times, but not *wrong*. I could work with difficult things. I didn't want out. All of us are tethered to life by love.

Ella and I needed each other and we were okay. Her small, warm body against mine. Her little face, covered in tears so quickly from the first wail. I know every single sound that leads up to crying when I hear her fall and bump her head on the table. I scoop her up to intercept the tears. Her legs clamping around me and her fists that clutch my shirt. I hold her on my hip, lean against the kitchen counter and talk to her in a low voice. She was born, she filled out, she lengthened, learned things, was deposited down on her feet, started to speak. She can't be left alone even for the duration of a shower or a bathroom visit. She can't open a door. She can't make a phone call. It's such a relief to have some time to myself when she's with Nick, but I think about her all the time anyway, like I'm lovesick. Her little mop of fluffed up silky, white hair on the top back of her beloved head. Her sticky little fingers that grab, her hot biscuit breath when she cries into my face. Her tiny, perfect teeth with a miniscule space between the two front ones.

As a child, I was always in the hospital—asthmatic, allergic to more and more things, wheezing, coughing, itching, always a bellyache for some reason or another. My tests results were always borderlining something dangerous that required more extensive testing to rule out. Somehow, though, Ella is amazingly—so far, knock on wood—in perfect health. I tell myself the only thing we know is this moment anyway, and even if everything were to go wrong, pediatric medicine has evolved a lot since the early '80s in Norway. My therapist once told me that it is common for pediatricians to fall out with parents, because they prioritize bonding with the children. That's not how it was with Dr. Simonsen. Certain things were done to me as a very young child that adults wouldn't be put through without general anesthesia these days. A needle of sedatives in my pale thigh while I sat in my mother's lap; an enormous machine that hung from the ceiling and Dr. Simonsen with the huge, black eyebrows standing by the bench, his white doctor's coat with the buttons right by my face in a darkened room. I tried to tell them to stop because I was retching, but soon discovered that my protests had no effect. Hands emerged to hold me down on the hard bench. Years of cooperation only to find that there never was any choice.

Afterwards, my mother wheeled me through the echoing corridors that connected the children's ward to the main hospital building in a stroller that belonged to the hospital, even though I was way too old, almost four.

On most occasions, I held my mother's hand. She was so stylish, with her Princess Di-style hair, her high-heeled tan boots and loose roll neck sweater. Walking down the hallways of shiny linoleum with the colored stripes, past the bathroom and the red sofas with the ragged children's books, the partitions of blonde lacquered wood, the statue of the lady with the baby. Straight into the room where Dr. Simonsen awaited, the large-eyed teddy bears with their hard, smiling doll faces and big stiff ears perched on the windowsill. I could see trees through the glass pane and there was a white cotton sheet on the examination bench. I preferred to climb onto the bench by myself with the help of a chair, rather than be lifted onto it. Afterwards they weighed me in my underwear. I always weighed less than they had hoped.

Sit spin: a spin done in a sitting position. The body is low to the ice, with the skating knee bent and the free leg extended.

The worst flare-up in months of my regular abdominal pain arrives through a night of bad sleep. I struggle through layers of shallow sleep, half-dreams riddled with endless administrative tasks to complete and ceaseless disapproval from the world. As always, the pain glows around my left side, a sinister mix of aching and nausea—not anywhere in particular that I can locate, though I grab my skin and press my palm into my side as if I could move it that way. When I lie on my back, the pressure of my weight against the bed is sore but lying on my side doesn't help. The pain level fluctuates from just below what requires some kind of action and a little worse than that. I can only take the minimum dosage of painkillers before work.

I can barely wait to leave my hot bed in the stuffy, tiny room but I also *need* to sleep. I know the day will be no better. There's clamor before dawn from the New York City trash trucks that have always seemed unnecessarily noisy. The morning feels never-ending, every step of our routine tiresome and quarrelsome. First, Ella undresses all the way down to her diaper while I have my back turned and am making breakfast so we have to start from scratch again. Then, just as we're about to leave, she runs back into the kitchen and spills juice all over herself so I have to wash the stickiness off her and change her shirt yet again. We have both shed tears before we say goodbye, though I hide mine from her, closing the bathroom door for thirty seconds while she howls at me to let her in.

Up the stairs and down. On the train, I notice myself keeping the cheerful commentary more or less going to Ella, even though I'm so drained that my voice is just a faint puff drawn from a shallow pint of air. A ghost of fatigue resembling a human being.

During my commute to work on the crowded subway after I've dropped Ella off, I'm so exhausted I actually consider asking a stranger for their seat. I look around at the shuttered faces around me, all of us swaying with the carriage as the noise ebbs and flows. Would anyone take pity on me? Not for the first time, I think to myself that a moment of desperate need is the worst possible time to have to ask for help. If I didn't need it, it would be no problem. If I were doing it on someone else's behalf, I would almost certainly be successful, full of confidence and righteousness. But I don't look like I need help—I look like a regular healthy person, just crankier and less attractive. Sometimes I wonder if there's something about my face when I'm in pain and struggling that makes people not want to help me. On those days, people seem to be less polite than usual, and I can't count on even the smallest courtesy.

I catch my reflection in the window of the subway car. My mouth is downturned, eyes dull and frantic. I look like I'm convinced that something horrible is about to happen, or like I'm about to start yelling in a desperate and high-pitched voice. If someone misunderstood my request or simply chose to be cruel, it would crush me. I just can't take that risk. I have to remain standing, folding in on myself and raking energy from the corners to get to work, running a private but familiar survival program in which I would sacrifice limbs to keep going.

I can't stop evaluating every surface as a potential place to rest. Even the speckled floor looks inviting at this point. It costs so much to stay standing, my body leaking energy with every sway and turn the train makes. I can't lean against the pole because of all the hands holding on to it. My midriff glows with nauseous, dull pain that seems to have turned up the volume the second I dropped off Ella. *Can I really not have the tiny amount of space my ass would take up on some surface in this city? Just a miniature shelf is all I need. I can't be this tired. Maybe I just can't hack this life on my own. Is my stomach ruined again? I have to get back on some serious endometriosis meds immediately. Why didn't I start the drugs right after Ella was born? What the fuck was I thinking, going with only hormonal birth control?*

Did I think I was some sort of regular person? I'm out of practice. Is this the new cyst I'm feeling? Or is there actually something new wrong with me? My whole life is just a story of things going wrong. Think only small thoughts for now. You felt alone in caring for Ella when you were with Nick, too.

Now at least I can do things the way I want. And he never was good on a day like this anyway. I would have been able to ask him to take Ella home, but it would have cost me. I would feel like his eyes were on me, keeping score. He would want to place himself in the middle of it and take control of the situation, without listening to me, without acknowledging the skill set I've acquired through my lifetime as a patient. It would require fighting, insisting, explaining—and still he wouldn't remember, the next time it came up. He would blame me for being irritable, for rationing my painkillers. It would come down to some kind of political issue, to the raw fact of our bodies alone in a room together, where I was simply unable to make him understand that living in mine, the way it is, isn't optional.

I have a lifetime of training in looking normal, in seeming like I'm not in enormous trouble. I'll get up the stairs. Then, rest a little on my feet because there are no benches anywhere in this city, unless you've already spent all your energy and walked all the way into a park, or that ridiculous set-up on Broadway where there are benches only on the center partition, with the cars rushing past on both sides as if daring you to try and relax. My purse takes a toll on my balance. *I should start using a backpack.* Then I just have to get through the station hall and down those blocks and into the elevator and down the corridor to my desk. Even if you can see where you're going, even if you're almost there, all these flat, straight streets, you still have to walk them. If someone could just help me. *Don't think about that now.*

If I can sit still for an hour or two, eat and drink something, I'll recharge, I'll be okay. Maybe I'll treat myself to a cab for one of the stretches home. *But it'll be rush hour, and too expensive.* I put in extra work hours on the days Ella's not with me, to have a little leeway for days like this. Luckily, I'm efficient and can cover a lot of ground when I'm feeling well. I've trained myself to stop wasting energy on being overly polite. I cannot afford to squander even a drop.

Will I raise Ella in a single stretch of gritted teeth survival mode? Will she ever even know a version of me that's not exhausted? Will I be the one she will blame for everything, the only one there? Will she remember me closing the door on her this morning? My brain whirring, I'm still on the train, still on my feet, still needing to lie down.

If there was something really wrong, I would have to let Nick have her. Would he even manage? He wouldn't allow me to take Ella to Norway. I let a moment of complete and utter miserable panic rush over me like a hot flash as the subway lights flicker off for a second.

I would be thrown back into my old element. *I would have to give up on making my life work.* There would be hospital rooms with their terrible, noisy Feng Shui and their ghosts of panics and agonies past. Vomiting in front of strangers. Needles through the skin, a million times. The weight of my drained body against the white hospital bedsheets. They would do everything they could to help me and that would only be about 40 percent of what I need. A miserable chill spreads through my chest. *What the fuck would I do? Can I really trust Nick to bring my daughter to see me? Could I let her see me sick and weak? How would her life be without me in it?* Her father would raise her too carelessly, without the attention to detail she needs. She would be an American through and through. *Who would tell her about me?* I would wash up like a corpse on the river bank of the Hudson with all the other unlucky people in this charming and merciless country.

All my strength, talents, and efforts that could do nothing in the end, solve nothing, lead nowhere. Caught again, caught forever, ruined, never getting away, everything gone. *Oh my God.*

I picture myself lying flat on my back on the floor of my apartment, just inside the closed front door, crying loudly—my throat fully opened to the skies to accommodate my hopeless grief. Misfortune towering over me like an old-fashioned knight about to sever my head once and for all.

That image feels good. Something in the top of my chest is soothed enough by it that I don't start crying right there. The train finally rattles into my stop and I get off.

Even as I get through the week and the pain slowly eases, I can't stop thinking of how things could go wrong. The fragile structures of our hopes and how unnecessarily thoroughly they're struck down. Our dreams could be wrecked a lot more easily anyway, with just a change in the air and light. The smallness of what we need—one more day of safety, another day of touching and talking to the people in our lives as if we have all the time in the world.

When I was in my mid-twenties, a friend of my sister and I named Elin succumbed to an exceptionally virulent type of cervical cancer that laid the land desolate in the course of just five months. She was pale and thin in photos taken during the months leading up to the diagnosis, but her doctors kept telling her to come back later, that it was just period pain. The cancer progressed unimpaired. She was taking classes at the university at the time, laughing with wine-stained teeth, discussing feminist tactics with the full expectation of seeing their effects on the world. She had long, straight, brown hair and sharp eyes that would not let you get away with any bullshit. Her laugh was loud. She had such courage and dignity at twenty-eight, much younger than I am now. The surgery at the start of her treatment included a hysterectomy and removal of her ovaries, which sent her straight into menopause. She gave an interview to the local paper about the case against her doctor, the one who failed to discover the cancer. She talked about how she had been raised not to question the authority of doctors and bitterly referenced Simone de Beauvoir's memoir when she said: "This is the story of a well-raised and dutiful young woman."

Elin was angry that the brochure they gave her about treatment only mentioned the effects on her sexuality in a few sentences addressed to a husband—angry at everyone who expressed concern about the loss of her ability to have children. "Are they fucking kidding me? Remove everything, just fix me!" None of it worked. Her piercing, terrified eyes in that photo that accompanied the article; her newly pronounced clavicles showing in an elegant, black, scoop neck top. She was buried in April.

I flash to myself falling and crushing Ella under me when I walk down subway stairs. I hold on to her hand hard on the platform. Cars screeching around corners and creepy-looking people on the train set off my anxiety, not to mention the possible implications of unfamiliar twinges in my stomach, or wondering if Ella is looking too pale and thin. I don't know how my parents survived all those years when I was in and out of hospital as a child, even though they were a nurse and a doctor. They managed, despite the pain of those memories for me. My mother, younger than I am now, alone in the room with respected doctors in the big city, would even dare to question their opinion when they wanted to redo testing yet again. People do what they have to, I guess. It can't be thought about. I just have to make one phone call home at a time and try to be present with them. Thinking of their pain in relation to mine is too much for my mind. I have to carry it elsewhere in my body—the back of my neck, perhaps. Or between the shoulder blades, where it stops my breath from drawing completely.

You can't always reach everyone. Even with your very best efforts, you can't always make yourself understood.

I take the subway to Ella's daycare and from there to work, retracing the journey on the way home. I don't have the luxury of being out of control. I want to be calm and collected. There are to-do lists, dinners to cook, healthy lunches to pack, insurance companies to deal with, physical therapy to attend, and the subway to go in and out of at least four times every day. A billion opportunities to not lose my cool when chaos threatens to take over. Shopping, laundry, the eternal cycle of adding and removing snacks and clothes from Ella's tiny backpack, the work of trying to close off our small life to trouble, not leaving even the smallest crack where it can get in.

One morning in the privacy of my cubicle, walls covered in Ella's drawings, I push away thoughts of Kjetil by finally creating an online dating profile. I'm only going to have a quick look anyway, so it won't matter what I call myself, but I spend more than a half hour trying to come up with a good username while keeping one ear on my boss, who's on the phone a few doors down.

Something makes me check all the boxes for what I'm "interested in": *Men*, *Women*, and *Casual*, although I haven't been on a date with a woman in ten years. It wasn't because I stopped finding women attractive, but the scope of my vision had narrowed somehow, along with everything else. Every situation seemed to have just one outcome.

After some doubt, I attach an old, blurry full-length photo I find in an old vacation email. I'm fairly sure my face isn't completely recognizable, much to my relief. I only write a few brief sentences about books and music.

Still, within the day, I receive messages from men who politely inquire about my day and my preferences in literature. It amazes me that none of them are crude. It seems the women on the site aren't going to run down my door without me making an effort, but men are just offering themselves up. I click through picture after picture of all these attractive young men I, in theory, could go out and meet as soon as I can get a babysitter. This is a much better idea than thinking about the past. There they are, displaying their tan, ripped stomachs at what seems to be an eternal barbecue chock-full of handsome men, laughing at the camera with beer glasses raised.

I lean close to the screen. *How much will I need to do to my body before I can show it to anyone?* Will a razor and a month of nightly Pilates in front of the TV be enough?

At physical therapy, I'm again installed under the hot packs on the plastic chair between two tables, my eyelids dipping. I listen to the goings-on in the clinic over the soundtrack of scratchy radio songs. A Latino man brings in a child-sized old lady with some kind of ski cap on her head. I wonder if she's his mother or grandmother. Either seems possible. They sit down in the half cubicle next to me. Chelsea takes down the woman's medical history. The old woman speaks in Spanish and the man translates. She recently had surgery on her arm and has at least one kind of cancer. I'm not sure if I hear the word "terminal". Both the man and the old woman seem passive and exhausted and it sounds like the man is only translating parts of what the old woman is saying. They're here to possibly relieve some of her pain after surgery. I hear Chelsea examining the woman, asking cheerful questions in her bright voice as if she didn't hear a word they said, as if it's irrelevant to her. Worse, it's as if she's there to somehow correct them, show them how to be less troublesome. Or am I projecting? I turn my head the other way, glad it's not me, not today.

As it is, water still boils. Oatmeal still swells. The neighbor's slim gray dog still jumps happily every time she sees us in the hallway, and Ella, who's a little scared of her, still greets her with a delighted, timid smile.

Cross-foot spin: An upright spin in which the skater gradually places the free foot behind the spinning foot and continues the spin on two feet with toes together.

Ella has been up since 5:30 a.m., moving through the apartment like a little chaos train, dropping off bunny rabbits, books, and small outfits wherever she goes. At one point, for ten wonderful minutes I lie back on the sofa while she arranges my hair like a fan against the fabric of the seatback. She stands next to me on the seat, and I hold on to her legs so she won't fall. She is completely absorbed, and I can admire the delicate precision of her small, serious face above me in peace. She is humming, and occasionally weaves a few real words and some made-up ones into a song that sounds vaguely familiar. I gaze at her round cheeks and rosebud mouth, her slender neck, how everything underneath her translucent skin is working and purring along perfectly and I experience a wave of happiness and immense gratitude that seems to fill the apartment like sunlight. *You and me.*

We leave for Nick's in the afternoon. I have an errand to do downtown so I've offered to drop her off for their weekend, but I'm also curious to see his place. He runs a business with two friends that seems to be doing well, some kind of software solution for real estate listings. His new apartment is not far from Chelsea Market. The doorman insists on calling him, even though I tell him we're expected. In the end, Nick's apartment turns out to be on the same floor as us, at the other end of a maze of carpeted floors.

Nick comes to the door as we arrive. Ella is quiet, but her eyes are twinkling and there's a huge smile on her face. She lets go of my hand, and as she rushes to him, there is a moment where the three of us are all smiling, our eyes almost a little too bright. *If this could have been hers*, I think. I quell the familiar bargaining monologue in my brain. Nick lifts her and swings her like a pendulum. Her coat rides up under his large hands around her small body, revealing her little diaper bottom inside her thin wool tights my mother sends from Norway. I'm slightly taken aback by how tall he is again. I can smell his fabric softener. I note his jawline when he laughs up at her. He is a good-looking man. His ash blond hair is getting a bit long, maybe starting to have a dash of gray in it. He is going to age well. Between the two of us, Ella could—in theory—emerge perfectly balanced in size and temperament. Not too large or too small, not too sensitive or too callous. Not too prone to tears, nor too prone to let herself off the hook too easily. When I think of it, I want her to have generous helpings of many of his traits—his tendency to be amused by the world, his confidence, entitlement, assuredness that he'll be seen and listened to. I loved his largeness when we first met. He seemed so solid. There was a time when he was always laughing and flinging me around too. Ella reaches for the ceiling when his arms are stretched out and her laugh almost creates a Doppler effect as he swings her low again.

He reenters the apartment still swinging a squealing Ella and I follow in the trail of their mingling laughter. The apartment has hardwood floors, a lot of gray tones, but only has windows on one short end. Everything looks new. It probably has excellent air conditioning to balance it, but, personally, I would rather live a lot more shabbily if I could have more natural light and air. It's quite stuffy in here. It's none of my business now how he spends his money, of course. It's a million times better that he's doing well than the opposite.

I pry my fingers off that line of thinking and force myself to shake loose and be an adult. *Everything is all right, Laura. Let it go.*

"Congrats on the new place. Pretty fancy."

"Thanks! Yeah, I got lucky."

I lean against the doorway of a standard New York kitchen, narrow and small with a sink and fridge on one side and a stove on the other. It's much prettier than my kitchen, mostly because everything is shiny and unused. The walls are painted gray, like the rest of the apartment. I'm relieved to see that I don't wish it were mine, though I would kill for a dishwasher.

"I had some people over last night for a housewarming of sorts."

"Did you have fun?" I hope I sound neutral.

"Yeah, yeah, everyone stayed late. I'm dragging a bit today."

I feel so tired, suddenly, and it'll be so long before I'm back at home to lie down. I usually dread my empty apartment after I drop her off, but I'm too exhausted for anything else. My shoulder hurts and I start rolling them. Does he know a lot of people I don't by now?

"How's work? Are your arms any better?"

"Fine...mostly fine. I just feel a bit overwhelmed lately. I'm getting physical therapy for my arms, though."

"Oh, how's that going?"

"Good, it's helping, I think. Or I think it will, but I've been having some pain so far..."

"Well, should you be doing it if it's making you worse?" He looks tired.

Ella has scampered off further into the apartment. *Why did I start talking about this?* He's already uncooperative about picking her up on the days I have physical therapy, and I don't want to give him ammunition against me. I really have to break the habit of telling him things as if they are still his business.

"Yeah, the physical therapist said these things often get worse before they get better. I've been ignoring the problem for a long time, so it does make sense." I stand up straighter, try to convey the posture of a competent woman who takes care of herself.

He folds his arms in front of his chest and leans against the wall across from me.

"Well, I don't know. If it's supposed to make you better... how much are you paying? Lord knows you can't afford for any more body parts to start malfunctioning. You're not exactly low-maintenance as it is."

I give him a death stare. He doesn't realize exactly what he's said, but he can tell he's stepped in something. Nick is prickly about "always getting into trouble" with me, "no matter what he says." *Does he think I'm unable to take care of his daughter?* I see myself through his eyes for a second, and I seem so fragile I can barely stand it. A new cyst. Well, fuck that. Half my life it looked like I was never going to be okay. But I'm still here, and I'm doing just fine.

"Jesus Christ, it's exactly because there isn't room for more trouble that I'm *taking care of this problem.*"

"What does your boss say about it? Aren't you missing days already?"

"She can't fire me. There's the Americans with Disabilities Act."

"But you're not disabled."

I have no idea if I would be covered under the ADA. Still, I continue, forcing myself to speak quietly since Ella is in the next room:

"What if I am? Even if *you* don't like the sound of it—it's not a choice. It's not difficult because I haven't figured out the best fucking way of doing it. *It just is difficult.*"

I didn't invent the difficulty of depending on people. It's not a personality flaw of mine. The message is everywhere. The air is saturated with it—independence and strength and pulling yourself up by your bootstraps (an image that is by its very nature impossible). "Take complete responsibility for your life," they say, as if the external forces don't matter at all. As if it all comes down to personal effort and attitude. As if money, support, and privilege had nothing to do with how your life turns out. As if what decides a sick or disabled person's fate isn't medical help, access, benefits and rights, but the ability to perform some arbitrary athletic act on a reality TV show. As if this, like everything else doesn't come down to money and power—do you have it or don't you? As if even if all these things were in place, it didn't take hard work just to maintain life, every day, for the rest of your life. As though, if you need help in any way, you owe it to the world to tap dance with a grin on your face for the rest of your days and supply photos they can superimpose their inspirational quotes over: "What's *your* excuse? The only disability in life is a bad attitude!" To always feel *blessed* and *grateful* despite your life consisting of endless pain, no deciding power over your own life, no privacy and having to rely on *people you did not choose* to help you out. To answer all invasive questions lightly and cheerfully. To pretend to not see the hatred that is so often right under the surface.

The rest of us have to find a way to live and try to enjoy our lives even if we are always on the outside, even if they don't even want to know about us. We have to find a way to live for and with each other, not them. To focus on where we can reach each other, not on those arenas where we will always, always lose. As long as we have enough support. Not all of it, but *enough*. As long as all your energy isn't lost before you can even start.

I wish someone would try to convince me to lean on them like they do on TV, with those speeches saying it's okay to rely on people. People chasing you down to confront you with your flaws in an interested and loving way, so they can tell you it'll all be fine and that "we're in it together." That has yet to happen in my life.

Still so caught up in how things look on TV. What am I, a child?

"So, you're just going to sue them when they fire you?"

"Fuck you, Nick."

I see him pulling himself together.

"Fine, fine. I'm sorry." He is stiff and angry. I've never gotten used to how apologizing is hardwired into Americans, and never know whether to take it at face value or as some hostile reflex, another way to fight. *The words are in place, what more do you want?* I don't respond. Once, in the middle of a fight, Nick yelled, "Jesus, why can you never ever apologize? Were you raised by wolves?" Maybe I was.

Nick starts to clear the dining table irritably. The table is cluttered with plastic cartons from Whole Foods and plastic glasses and plates from plastic packaging marked *Extra Heavy-Duty*. Why should anything disposable be extra heavy-duty? I can see actual glasses through the open cupboard door. *Why didn't he simply use the glasses he owns instead of plastic? There's even a dishwasher!* This lazy extravagance used to infuriate me when we lived together. That American boy thing, seeing the world as a place opulent with things that are his to use up and not even recycle—almost as if there's virtue in it, like being thrifty never occurred to him because he's so wealthily innocent. He would say "Relax, honey!" wide-eyed, like he really had no idea why I would bruise his easy, happy way of being in the world. *There's always been enough of everything for him.* I can still sense that line from ten feet away—where his attention and fondness for me ran out in favor of "being reasonable", of there being limits to what I could ask, how weird I could be, how much I could need from him.

It's so hard to watch the person you love be in pain. It's a natural impulse to want to fix it, and not being able to is uncomfortable. Remaining in that state of discomfort over time is even harder. Being in a relationship with someone in chronic pain is like a chronic pain condition in and of itself.

At times, it strikes me as a sort of fair deal that I let go of Kjetil's seemingly boundless acceptance of me and my limitations to end up with this: a fairly kind, normal man, whose heart held limited portions of everything when it came to me. Someone who, in the end, needed me to be different from who I am. It was a natural result, in a way. When Nick and I met, I was so concerned with my own privacy and an idea of how to be an adult New Yorker—*keep your secrets and your pain to yourself.* I talked to some of my friends about my health, but took enormous comfort in how untroubled I could appear with Nick and others. I was caught up in his burly, cheerful ways, his manner of turning everything into a joke. His handsome largeness and rude health seemed to come from a more solid, brighter, easier world than I did. I wanted in—badly.

In time though, that lighter world came to feel how certain American buildings feel to a European: an imitation curiously lacking in detail, everything a little too large. I came to see that our lives are not the same, aren't even similar. Things are different for a tall, handsome, healthy man. All the ties that bound us were dissolvable—but one.

Before I leave, Nick and I patch things up, more or less.

I call out for Ella, but she doesn't come and I go into the living room to say goodbye. She's on the floor, absorbed in playing with her bunny and a doll I haven't seen before. My body needs hers. All I want is to lift her up and breathe in the scent of her, but I resist, knowing it will only make my departure more difficult. I settle for bending down and kissing her hair.

The mixture of heartbreak and relief I feel when I leave…

I walk outside and the cold air feels so good. New York City is enormous, dark, and empty around me. The city noise echoing down the blocks and up the walls into the falling dusk. Inside Nick's apartment, the two of them play and cuddle and hum and laugh, those warm bodies that I know so well. And I'm heading elsewhere, alone.

I was quite old before I first realized people say hurtful things to me because they care and that it's difficult for them to see me in pain. Since it hurts to face the situation head-on, it's tempting for them to believe I'm at fault rather than accept that often, when it comes to my health, the situation sucks no matter what I do. The pain is here; a certain damage has been done and cannot be undone. People sometimes prefer to believe that I'm failing to follow their advice and making mistakes they can judge me for, rather than accepting that I'm suffering. This shields them from the full weight of being present and offering support, even when they can't fix anything. I feel as if they're telling me I'm somehow wrong and therefore don't have a right to suffer, or to talk about it, maybe even to exist. Maybe their actual message is: *Please stop. I can't stand my part in this. I can't stand to witness the relentlessness of your pain.*

The further out on the fringes you are, the further from regular people's lives, the more you are blamed for your troubles. You'd think that if things get very, very bad, there would be support—allowances, and understanding and love like you've always wanted. But it's not true. When things get very bad, people often pull away. They and their reassuring friends have no problem finding sensible reasons for detaching themselves.

When it came to my parents, I suppose they believed it was necessary to keep me striving no matter what. The situation was not hopeless, because my mother could always produce some way that I should have known better or could have acted better to avoid getting sick. There was no need to panic, because the next time it would be different. Pretending my health was in my power and not so bad anyway may have been necessary for our survival, but it was still less than ideal for the most vulnerable party—me.

As a parent, even one who hasn't been severely tested yet, I can see that the opportunities to make mistakes are staggering.

The time before I left Norway is a vaguely remembered miserable fog. Many women have similar stories, and it's not as special to me as I thought back then. Still, my experiences as a constantly sick child prepared me in the worst possible way for the situation. Thinking nothing could be done anyway, I went with my basic programming and ignored the symptoms until my endometriosis was a hideous stage-four mess that had taken over my pelvis and abdomen and left me twisted with pain. Even though I had been brushed off by doctors many times when I had brought up my symptoms, even though I'd called and called to try to move up appointments and surgery dates, it felt as if there was something ugly in not having done more to protect myself—in clearly thinking it was okay—normal—for me to be in such pain. It felt disgusting, like I had done it to myself. I'd acted stupidly on instinct, like an animal, as if I was trying to hide and die instead of getting treatment and owning my life, the limited way it was available. I'd been trying so hard to act as if I was normal that I allowed the tiny space that was actually mine, all 110 pounds of human flesh, to be ruined.

Occasionally, Kjetil and I would exchange some desperately hopeful words about things getting better eventually—but my real path to survival, which was getting the fuck out of there, was going to squeeze him out of my life. During one of many dark nights, Kjetil and I stood on each side of the kitchen table under fluorescent lights, with my stomach on display between us because it hurt too much to have even the lightest of fabrics covering it. The second I got in the door, I had to pull down the soft waistband of the yoga pants I was wearing below my hip bones, so they wouldn't pain me as much. But it was the coldest winter in years and there was no way to solve it; I was always cold and in pain.

My stomach stuck out like I was pregnant, although they told me I could probably kiss ever being pregnant goodbye. I was sobbing, as usual, my arms clutching each other over my stomach, and it wasn't some theoretical question of what I might've been doing to him: we were both choking on the despair filling our apartment. I couldn't tell you how the nights ended up like this, they just did. There would be a flare of frantic rage and later we would hold on to each other desperately. I'd drug myself to get a few hours of fitful sleep and wake up the minute the drugs ran out . I was trying, like any patient in desperate need, to take only what was given and not demand more. I *never* got let off easily. I couldn't grit my teeth and get past this, I couldn't change it. My exposure made me furious.

I worked myself into a froth listing everything that was horrible until I cried. I said things like: "Everything is ruined. They just Scotch-taped me together to hobble along until I die. All I've ever fucking done is behave and now it's too late to do anything else, I can't have a normal life and I can't go to New York either, I can't do anything, I can't have *anything*."

He sighed. "It'll be okay."

"It will not be okay! It will so thoroughly, profoundly not be okay. And you know it, you just want me to shut up about it. You might as well just tell me to shut up."

"I don't want you to shut up."

"You do, look at you! You're sick of me."

He was upset, too, but he could always keep his voice calm.

"Of course, I'm sick of the situation, but I'm listening to you. I just don't see what good will come of dwelling on everything that's negative."

"Well, what should I be dwelling on then? Am I supposed to just sit inside this apartment and puke and take painkillers until I die? I should just kill myself."

"I get it, okay? But I'm on your side! We're in this together."

But he looked so exhausted. What was he really thinking? His crushed eyes, his frown. His tears that came so easily, like it never occurred to him that something bad could come of showing vulnerability.

I sobbed. "But you can *leave* if you want to, and you can sleep through the night, and people leave your fucking body cavities alone, and you're not in pain every second of every fucking day! So don't tell me that we're in this together." I was both testing him and pushing him away, but even now, there is no insight I've gained that would have changed it.

When I left, I figured Kjetil would date a tall lawyer or economist with earning power and a strong, fertile body and a happy family to match his. I pictured his life without me as a TV commercial where people throw Frisbees, host pretty dinner parties, and enjoy tidy, able lives with no trouble, ever. I felt like it was a favor to him that I excised myself from his life—I was heavier than I had any right to be, toxic like mold. This thought brought anger, too, it was a matted, dirty mess. I felt I had no choice.

On Sunday afternoon, I have my headphones on while doing the dishes and a young woman on the Norwegian public radio podcast refers to oral sex as "the figure skating of the sex Olympics." She has a loud, endearing laugh and leads a regular feature about sex, talking with ease about specific sexual how-to's in a way that would never air in the US. I would have died of embarrassment to hear it when I was in the program's intended age range for listeners.

I was a teenage figure skater. Maybe because she isn't the flawless apparition of an Olympic athlete on TV—just a young, Norwegian voice in my ears—the notion of skating sticks in my head. The American skaters always look so put-together, their makeup perfect. I love to watch them, but I have much more tender feelings towards the Eastern European girls, who sometimes have bad teeth, or wear a slightly off shade of concealer, or too-bright hair clips that could've easily been hidden if anyone had thought to.

I check where I think my old skates might be, on the top shelf in the back of the hallway closet. I have some energy, so when they happen to be right there, I put a coat on, shove the skates in a Paris Review tote bag, and head out the door.

I find myself in a seat in the nearly empty subway car rattling towards the skating rink only twenty minutes after the thought even occurred to me. It's late, and I haven't even checked if the rink is still open. All the way there I try to persuade myself that *it's no big deal*, just because I haven't skated at all in ten years, it doesn't matter, I don't have anything better to do with my Ella-less night. I listen to music and feel fairly relaxed, but when I get off the subway and start walking over to the rink—four long, deserted blocks—there is no cool left. I hurry and pray for the universe to give me a break, just this once—please, *please* let nothing get between me and the ice.

I think of all those times when I was a kid, waiting for the bus, then walking all the way around the little lake and up all those hills to the rink, only to find it closed—why did that happen so often? I used to call the rink to try and make sure it was open, but you couldn't be sure it was closed just because no one picked up. It was pre-internet. The disappointment was so harsh that I can still feel it.

Of course, when I get to the rink, it is closed. I've never been inside before, but instead of searching for the public entrance, I walk through the open industrial-looking door by a pile of rink-snow. I'm free to walk all the way up to the boards, breathing in the clean, slightly chemical ice, but there's no one here. *Why did I leave so late?* I don't even know why I brought the skates from Norway, spent that valuable suitcase weight years ago that I could have otherwise spent on *kaviar* tubes, *Jordan* toothbrushes and tins of *Stabburet* mackerel in tomato sauce.

I lean against the boards and feel tears prick my eyes.

Just then, a bald Asian man in his sixties wearing work clothes comes through the door of what looks to be a changing room. I brace myself to be told to vacate the premises. Instead, he takes one look at my face and takes pity on me.

"You really, really want to skate, huh? You know, we're closed."

He pauses for effect.

"What the hell, I can give you twenty minutes."

"Really?"

"I have to finish up in there anyway," he says, gesturing to the changing room. "Twenty-five minutes at the most. Don't make me regret it."

He smiles when he sees I have tears in my eyes. I thank him profusely, but he just waves it off before disappearing into a back room. Sometimes, New York is a miraculously generous city.

I hurry to put my stuff on the bench and shrug off my coat, kicking off my boots at the same time. I insert my feet into the reassuring, stiff, padded leather of my skates that my parents spent so much money on when I was thirteen, bought with space to grow into. I lace them up tightly, my hands shaking. My arms remember perfectly how to unsheathe the blades from their plastic protectors in a single movement.

I put my earbuds in, my gloves on, and then I carefully step out of the gate on to the ice. *Ah...* The ice is rough, so I keep an eye on it for treacherous grooves. I can't risk a fall. I carefully glide for a few strokes, listen to the soft *crr crr* of the incisions. The joy is immediate. *This!*

I start building up a little more speed, circling the rink to warm up like I used to, only more slowly. When I hit the short end of the rink, I start to cross over carefully, but my speed is still much faster than running, only with so little effort. The smooth glide over the ice feels wonderful and my body calls the shots, carefully teaching itself to skate again. My toes are a bit pinched and my skates aren't laced tightly enough, but muscles on the outside of the back of the thighs and buttocks engage and keep me steady.

Without thinking about it, I flip from the outer edge forwards to the inner edge backwards and start crossing over that way. My playlist is full of young bands that nevertheless have a dreamy '80s or '90s style. A woman's clear voice with a warm lift and space in it translates itself automatically to the kind of dance-y moves that go with skating, the long glides and turns. This music has been calling out for the movements of skating all along. Anything I could do on two feet would be clumsy and staccato by comparison.

I turn up the music and let myself do it—dance on the ice. I feel so good I half want an audience to share this with, but no one is there. Even the man is out of sight.

Not that it would be impressive to watch anyway, mostly turns and crossing over and of course the music is inside my headphones, but the small ways I dance to the music make me feel magical, young, new. It's mine and mine alone. I have the entire rink and I remind myself to enjoy it, that I'm not likely to get the ice to myself ever again. Fourteen-year-old Laura would have peed her pants with joy at the thought of having a rink to herself—in New York City, of all places—and the ability to listen to any music she wanted while skating.

I skate backwards and start building up spccd in a smaller circle. My body has its own ideas of what we're doing. I allow it a careful pirouette, gathering speed with my arms. I'm spinning on the blade of one skate, my hair flying straight out with the velocity, keeping the pick of the other one touching the ice for safety.

When the pirouette ends, I'm dizzy and almost fall, even though it's fewer than half the turns I used to be able to do. No elegant exit on one foot with my hands hip-height and my face upturned, just slowing down and stabilizing myself with both feet, my heart suddenly pounding with the terror of falling. *What if I broke something?*

As my heart rate settles, I admire the circles I've carved in the ice. Impressively little wandering considering how long it's been.

When I leave the ice after twenty-two minutes, I'm shaking. For some reason, my back hurts on the right side, down towards my hip. My leather boots are floppy, loose, and too light; my steps stubby and lumbering.

I'm as worn out as a dishrag, and I'm happy.

The lightness lasts beyond the weekend. On my way home after a full day of work, I wait for a light to change in the roar of Midtown traffic. Steam rises from the street and I let myself experience the crowd as an embrace, rather than a crush. As the light changes and I start to make my way across the street, my eyes rest on a small cluster of suit-clad men outside an office building. I stop breathing before I have time to think.

There is no way.

One of the men looks like Kjetil. Am I losing my mind? But my entire body responds to his familiar silhouette. I pause for a moment until a car honks its horn at me and I hurry on to the other side, at which point possibly-Kjetil turns his head and spots me. *It's him.* I freeze in my tracks. *Shit.* He, too, is frozen, his face stricken. I half want to turn on my heel and run for my life. I watch him start to excuse himself awkwardly from the other suit-wearing men. It's been six years since we last saw each other.

His face looks a little more lined, and he's too thin, like he's been distilled into an essence of himself. He's always been beautiful, in a way that takes a little time to notice—his warm, brown eyes, his lovely hands, the straight, broad brushstrokes of his dark eyebrows. I quickly take stock of myself. I'm glad I put on lipstick before I left the office. My navy trench coat is flattering and in good shape, and I'm wearing a red patterned scarf that goes well with it. I may look a little worse than I did four years ago, but look better than I did six years ago when Kjetil last saw me. *Thank God.* I'm clenching my jaw and my fists in my pockets and I'm almost gasping for breath.

No sign of his trademark happy, generous smile that reveals his slightly crooked teeth now. He's dressed a little too fashionably, more than he used to be. He didn't use to look that comfortable wearing a suit. His black hair is short and sharp, as always, but the front is pulled over to one side in a new way. He doesn't look out of place in New York, but he also doesn't quite look like a finance guy. Maybe it's the suit, how it fits him more snugly than his colleagues', or maybe it's his hair, but there's something strangely foreign and almost a tiny bit effeminate about him.

Here I am, reading him like some American would.

I force myself to take a deep breath in through my nose and out through my mouth.

Do I want to hear what he might have to say to me? He doesn't look like he even wants to talk. Maybe I should just go? What would he do if I just took off running down the street?

He reaches me. I feel my eyebrows lift and I open my mouth, unable to get a word out. I realize that I'm smiling. Despite everything, it seems I'm happy to see him.

"Hei!"

"Hei!" We clumsily move towards each other, not sure how to act, and hug briefly. His cold cheek brushes mine. He smells of fresh air.

"Oh my God, it's you," I blurt out. "So good to see you." It's an Anglicism, my Norwegian is a little rusty. I blather on: "Can you say that in Norwegian?" *Shut up Laura.*

"Yeah, good to see you, too." He's smiling, but it looks a bit strained. Should I pretend I don't know why he's here? That he's divorced? No, it's awkward enough.

"Do you live here, now?"

My arms squeeze against my body and I've become a stiff, tense little stem for my up-tilted face, which is smiling broadly up at him, hopefully keeping appearances up for all of us.

"Yeah, I work here, in there, actually." He gestures towards a glass and concrete tower lit up with office windows, just like the ones around us. I'll never get used to this part of Manhattan. I'm still as thrilled and oppressed by it as any tourist. A bus passes and the noise makes us draw closer to the wall. It's almost dusk. Regular life is going on elsewhere. Nick is probably brushing Ella's teeth by now, Ella sitting on his knee with his leg up on the toilet in his new, bright bathroom, while he sings and makes her laugh. She's probably trying to hold on to the toothbrush over his hand and puckering her lips around the head of it.

"How is it?" I'm tilting my head, still smiling and I feel my eyes crinkle, looking up at him. Am I actually flirting? *Jesus Christ.*

He smiles. His eyes are cool, polite.

"Hard. Absurd amounts of work. But it'll be fun, I think." He looks towards the building when he talks about work. "They keep calling me 'Kah-jaytil'." He adds.

I laugh. "Maybe you'll have to drop the J? Ketil? That would make you 'kettle,' I guess."

He laughs a little, too. I shift from one foot to another.

"Yeah, now that it's been a little while, it's 'Chaytil', which is good enough. Ah, I don't know! Maybe I'm just jet-lagged. I feel a little weird, actually. It takes so much energy to talk and smile and be on my best behavior at all times. To act like a human being around all these Americans."

We both laugh nervously.

"I know," I say, nodding. "In the beginning here, I didn't know which way was up."

"I seem to remember." And just like that, we're in dangerous territory. He gives me a little smile, but he doesn't look like he has many more smiles saved up for me. His eyes are so grave. I always hated to see him sad. It feels as if we're still trying to reach each other. As if we're still each other's business. *How close to the surface this is for both of us.*

Ten minutes ago, I was heading home to spend a safe and relaxing evening with my TV. *What have these years been like for him?* His face is serious and tired. *What the hell am I doing? I have to get out of here. I'm not ready to hear what he might say.* I try to change the subject.

"So...what made you leave Norway in the end?"

"Well, the opportunity presented itself, and it was time for a change. It hasn't been a good year, let me put it that way. I got divorced."

"Hey, me too." I smile and blush.

"Fun stuff, isn't it?" He returns my smile.

"The best."

"Time of my life."

"Just makes you feel so good about yourself, you know?"

"Brings out the best in everyone. Such an atmosphere of forgiveness and love."

We both laugh. The neat shoulders of his suit. The short black hair near his left temple, where the small scar I know so well mars the blackness with a faint, white half-moon.

"Oh, wow. I'm so jetlagged, still." He raises his eyebrows and exhales heavily. "How strange to see you."

My stomach drops.

"I know."

Please don't ruin all those tender memories.

"And good. I've missed you."

"You have?"

"Yeah."

Am I really going to say something?

"I guess I thought I mostly made everything more messed up for you," I say.

He shrugs. "You left me."

It's a lightning bolt of realization that is years late. His dark eyes, so sincere. *He did love me. And I left.*

I don't know what to say. Is it shame I'm feeling?

We walk to the subway together. It's only a block and a half, disappointingly short, but also a relief. He lives in Brooklyn. We make conversation about New York neighborhoods. I tell him about Ella and he laughs at my stories about her. We don't make plans to see each other. We just hug again and say goodbye, and I feel him holding on to me for a few seconds longer than necessary. His cold ear against my cheek again. I breathe in his scent—a new cologne, yet familiar. I'm still surprised at his older, narrower face when the embrace ends. I watch him pour down the subway stairs.

On the way home, I realize I'm absolutely spent. I manage to capture a seat on the express train, and as I close my eyes and lean my head against the wall, there's a sense of release. It felt good to be seen by those eyes after all these years. There are other parts of me than what I've experienced in the past six years. *The past wasn't all painful.* I could see him again.

When I left Norway, I needed my misfortune to be my business and mine alone. I hadn't yet decided whether I could live with it. Maybe I just wanted to get out of there, too. Maybe it doesn't make sense, maybe escaping was just what I wanted. There was no tidy arc, no lesson learned that can fit neatly in the lock and open everything, make it all okay or worth it.

Perhaps I would have a better life if I could manufacture more meaning from it all. Through illness, you mostly just get screwed. You lose so much time, putting in full days of misery and there is really no end to how bad it can get. Time spent suffering didn't teach me anything I wanted to learn. But perhaps as time passes, it's possible to learn not to blame yourself. Life is hard enough. Take what is offered, because it might not always be around. You can't be harder and harder, stronger and stronger, more and more disciplined until you compress into a diamond. People aren't mineral or metal. They are soft flesh, where love and pain echo through the body. Sometimes you have to ease up, to let go. You never know what will be able to help you. Compassion and gentleness are also endless.

There are limitless possibilities inside other people. They could possibly say something other than what you expected.

I leave work early for physical therapy before I pick up Ella. My lower back is still sore from skating. After the first half of the session, which includes the electric stimulation, hot packs, ultrasound, and a little massage, Chelsea leads me to a small cluttered room.

"I think the traction machine might work for you," she says. It's fastened to one end of the massage table and has chains and hooks and a long arm of some kind. It resembles something children with tuberculosis were tortured with in the '40s.

Chelsea instructs me to lie down on my back and tightens a wooden brace around the back of my neck. When she fastens a strap across my forehead, I try not to tense up. She gives me an emergency stop button, starts the machine and turns off the light as she leaves. It starts to whir.

The window behind my head illuminates the room faintly. The knuckles on my right hand brush against the cool wall. It feels familiar though I've never been in this room before. It occurs to me that every Norwegian doctor's office is arranged like this and that I must have been in this exact position in a room, on an examination table up against the wall, headboard towards the window, many times. Weakened in some way and left to recover alone for a minute while the nurses wondered what to do with me.

As the machine whirs ominously, I wonder if it's a specific unpleasant memory that's tugging at me, and whether it will be an ordeal to lie here alone in a dark room for ten minutes. Suddenly, the traction machine starts its work. I blink nervously at the ceiling as it lifts the brace around my neck and stretches my neck gently, more evenly and calmly than any human hands could. It relieves a pressure I wasn't even aware of, it's been there for so long. The small muscles that tie the back of my skull to my neck, now softened and tender from the massage and heat pack after being hardened nuggets for so long, are slowly released. Every time the brace lifts my head I experience an intense relief. It feels so good to have my head out of my hands for a minute.

The machine puts it down, sore and heavy, then lifts it gently. I am being taken care of.

When I leave, something has been rearranged. I can stand up straight. I can move my head eight new different directions. I can tilt it without compensating with my entire neck. My head feels so loose it almost seems dangerous. I feel two inches taller—literally.

Spins: continuing turns pivoting on a blade that does not leave the ice.

For days I feel dizzy and strange, like something huge has shifted. My neck is tender. I expect it to tighten up any day, to go back to being impossible to straighten properly, but it stays loose. At work and in the mirror at home, I keep noticing that my posture is straighter, my face looks different—better. It used to look like that a long time ago.

I want to try on clothes and put on makeup. Tiny spaces reappear between each rib, between my lower ribs and breasts in particular. Space emerges between the collarbones and the neck. My neck itself lengthens upwards. I can draw a full breath easily, straight into the entire area between my eyebrows and pelvis, like a gust of wind. There's a husk of grief I just might shake off. I want to be free of it all. I want a wave to come crashing down on every old pattern—leaving only soft sand where there were once hard calluses, calcified and fossilized.

After Ella's bath, she's in her chair at the kitchen table while I'm spreading avocado on a slice of bread, her *kveldsmat*. The soft light over the stove makes my shabby old kitchen look prettier than it actually is. The half-lit kitchen with the hum of the refrigerator reminds me of being a child myself. Clean cotton pajamas that dried in the fresh air on the line behind the house, with nicely stuck-together sleeves that parted crisply for my arms as I held them up for my mother to pull my PJ top over my head. Eating and babbling under the gaze of a thoughtful and tired adult, feeling the damp silky hair against my cheeks and neck, and being tucked into bed.

Years ago, I read a *Time* magazine feature about chronic pain sufferers and how new treatments like antidepressants and meditation can help. Some of the interviewees were born with illnesses that caused pain, so they'd been living with it for years. There was a picture of a boy on a bed in his resting cubicle, which had been installed in his high school's bathroom. The *Time* journalist commended the school for the adjustments they made, the effort they put in for this particular boy. In the photo, his wheelchair was parked next to the sink. It didn't seem like a prize to me, to spend an extra hour a day in the boys' bathroom.

There was also a woman in her early forties who had led a completely regular life—until one day, a huge metal filing cabinet fell on her out of nowhere at work. After that, every moment of her life was crisscrossed with black scrawls of excruciating pain from damaged nerves in her spine. It never went away. Surely when that happened, you would look back and think that everything before that moment was blessed, perfect. That nothing could've possibly been wrong enough to not lie around smiling like a cat in a spot of sunshine, as long as your body wasn't firing more and more pain at you. Any day that a filing cabinet doesn't fall on you. Life only has to be good *enough*.

"Mamma! Se på meg! Look!"

I haven't taught Ella to speak Norwegian fluently, but a few words have stuck. I should teach her, so she can talk to her cousins. *I should take her home to meet them, too.*

"Mamma mamma mamma!"

My daughter grins at me, displaying her pearly teeth with a little avocado smeared around her mouth. Her white-blonde hair fluffs up unevenly like a little chicken's, like mine did when I was her age. She has threaded crayons in between her fingers, and she's twisting them in slow jazz hands. My healthy daughter in our clean kitchen on a regular evening, no one coming and no disaster imminent. *Knock on wood.* I can work with this.

PART 2

YOU ARE HERE

2013

New York has a good effect on me. For three years, I've been getting better and better at life. I've graduated and started working at Scandinavia House a few months ago. Nick and I work and exercise and go to parties, events, museums. I'm amazed at all I can do. I only have time to write on the weekends and on the subway, but it feels so good to have a proper job. I'm going to start sending my stories out soon.

If I can just keep moving I will always be all right. Everything that's not here right now, I can do without. It's all about keeping my eyes on the target, up on that high story where we've climbed, where the light spills onto the smooth floor. Where things are what they are, clean and free of dark thoughts. Those thoughts can be put away and the situation will be exactly the same, only better. I am not ruined yet.

It's a little like being drunk. Dizziness leads to carelessness, which leads to the delicious discovery that I will be okay, even when I take chances. I won't be hit by a car because I dash across the road; I won't die from eating a French fry without inquiring in the perfect way about the ingredients.

Not that I'm careless much—I'm still trying to stay ahead of the curve—but I'm much more of a normal person in New York than I ever was in Norway. I can solve some of the problems of bad health and lack of energy easily—cabs are cheap and plentiful here and I can order allergy-safe food to my door twenty-four hours a day, seven days a week. There are moments of shortness of breath as I try to thread the things I need to get done ever more tightly through the days, as if I can eliminate the loss of even the smallest bit of energy—and then I would look even more like a New Yorker, lean and tightly wound and always with something a little too eloquent on the tip of my tongue from all that time on the subway reading in between conversations. Conversations never run out in New York, there's always so much to tell and discuss. Sparks fly.

New York crushes in on even my modest life, making it louder and more exciting, more pressure, more of everything, a wonderful spasm of sorts. My breath is more urgent. I snatch a little rest here and there and then get caught up all over again. I use every last scrap of myself.

Writing at my desk, I feel that same rush of heat and noise and diffuse myself in it like a teabag in a big, white cup. It's glorious to not have to hold everything inside for a little while. As if I can levitate off the ground just a little, privately, through minute mastery, like the first time I managed a little yoga lift. Placing my hands between my more or less lotused legs and my body, and realizing I can defy gravity by tightening my core muscles and turn into the bud of a peony, a ball on top of a tiny stem. I can levitate out of the traffic jam of trouble that so often has been my life. Hovering and slowing down the space between the moments of complete terror. *This moment is okay, and this one, and this one, too.* This one spills sunshine on my face; this one, a soft, warm breeze. This one is crisp piano music drifting from the speakers; and now, an unbroken string of words typed by my fingers. A balance of effort, discipline, surrender, and release.

Lifts: the lifts are just as they sound: pairs elements in which the man hoists his partner above his head with one or both arms fully extended. The lift consists of ascending, rotating and descending movements that define the lift.

Nick is tall and fair, a giant compared to me. I'm almost embarrassed to walk on the streets with another blond in this city teeming with gloriously diverse beauties. He is cheerful and likes to make fun of me. With him, it's easy to focus on what's going well. I feel low at times, but he never does. We got married at the courthouse a month ago, without telling anyone besides a few friends. Apart from everything else, it helps with my immigration status.

Nick was a football player in high school and is still in shape at thirty-three. He could carry me all day long, literally. He would be useful to have on my side in the zombie apocalypse. His hands are big. His shoulders are wide. All day long I long to be reunited with his body—his large, warm embrace and his perfume (clean but also spicy and full of heat). When I smell him, I get that feeling I did as a child, that a scent could hold secret worlds where everything was different; better and more profound. Maybe those worlds are memories of other lives just as good as this one, other eyes to look through—a million brief, private experiences that are impossible to share.

Nick's un-curious head above it all, not asking questions. He is familiar but deeply exotic to me, just like this city, this country. I love him, but there are certain things I might never truly understand about what drives him, what undoes him. His body speaks more eloquently than he does. He is tender and okay with being careful. He leaves me in peace. He, like this incarnation of me, keeps all his shit on his side of the line, like a good American. *Be proud of your shit, own it, and don't let it get on other people.*

He doesn't care what I do for a living. He is funny in a general TV and internet-based way: somewhat to the left of mainstream culture, all about being well-informed. He is always trying to find things to laugh at. He has a rude sense of humor and I always giggle when I'm with him, past the point where I normally would contribute something funny to the conversation myself. I am consuming him, swallowing him down like he is delicious food. I keep my eyes on him.

It's a relief that all he has to do to avoid my allergic reactions is wash his face, hands, and brush his teeth carefully before kissing me. He would probably do that anyway—at least brush his teeth. He is always flossing and rinsing out his mouth with mouthwash. A fear of smelling bad is programmed deep in him. Americans shower so much and always shroud themselves in scented products. A New York subway car containing homeless people still often smells cleaner than a regular rush hour tram in Oslo. Don't get me started on France.

We don't actually spend much time together compared to my previous relationships. He works long hours and I like to have time to myself in the apartment to write. We don't share that many meals. I don't usually join him to eat in restaurants, except for a few sushi places I trust, but it's okay. I can cook my own food and meet him later.

He's not looking too hard at me, not overthinking anything.

He seems happy.

His actual body as an object: his sweat tastes bitter and salty like anyone's, though his sweat smells sort of fresh to me. How strange it is that a body is as much a body in this country as it is at home. As if I wasn't aware of that before I had slept with a citizen. Equally covered in skin, which has pores and hairs when you get up close, as heavy on the ground, stinking out his socks, wearing out his pants in the crotch and knees, buying toilet paper, chewing. His body, fed on GMO corn, hormone-laced eggs and milk all his life, is constructed from different material, from plants I don't know the names of, from other strains of grains, his body is almost exclusively created from food that could kill me. Grown in this newer nation with its softer, more savory air, a handsome white boy with a large, strong, fast body, he has always been seen, always acknowledged.

It turns out taking what the body wants can be easy. At a friend's party in Crown Heights, I admired him across the room for a while before approaching him. I have always been a sucker for beauty. I was tipsy and happy with my kimono-style silk top. I kept having great conversations with everyone I talked to. I reflected to myself that my appreciation for his simple brand of masculinity had come with age. I never had a taste for it when I was younger, but it seemed as I was getting older I could enjoy more kinds of beauty in a wider range of people.

There was a certain heaviness in his well-built body. Sleepy eyes, a little small for the planes of his face, a trace of his Eastern European heritage. He was sitting on the low sill of a dark window with a view of Manhattan, at ease, as always. I was telling him about graduate school when he shifted his body and moved one of his long, jeans-clad legs so that his foot rested just between my toes. I lifted my eyes to his and smiled. I didn't even blush.

I had barely touched another person in years, except for hugging friends and leaning on them when I was drunk. It was a hot night, which made me relax. We left the party early and went straight to his apartment. On his bed, with only a small lamp lit, uncovering it part by part, I found his body deeply appealing. I hardly thought of Kjetil at all. Lying on his back, Nick arched his neck and closed his eyes, like he was surrendering to me. While he was getting a condom from his nightstand, his back to me, I stared at the ceiling and tried to figure out how to give him a few directions for my small, sore body. It felt vital to tell him, to force the situation to be good, so I could be present and not just go silent and wait it out. But I wanted more than anything to not have to say anything.

"Go *really* slow at first, okay? Don't touch my stomach except very softly or it will hurt."

"Okay," is all he said, smiled and moved his glorious nakedness back across the bed towards me with care.

The taste of red wine in his mouth when we kissed, his dick in latex between my legs like any other, hardness and softness, figuring out how to cooperate, how to connect, how to spread waves of sensation into the other person's body. It felt known yet new. It felt good. He is a straight man but has slept around a lot; he takes direction well and knows his stuff. I appreciated how it felt almost like the queer experiences of my past, like any two bodies figuring out how to tease pleasure out of each other, without taking for granted that the other person will enjoy what the last one did or even have the same parts. With his mouth on my neck, I felt intoxicated by so much warm skin against mine.

He had awakened a robust and healthy-feeling lust in me that I was thrilled to encounter again, for the first time in years. It made things easier. One moment, on my back underneath him, it felt impossible. But the next moment, it was fine, sexy, dirty, almost like something I could do without thinking, without worrying. He moved carefully and intentionally. As the heat built between us and he was less careful I liked that, too. I had lots of practice in reworking pain: relaxing, leaning in, leaning out, finding pleasure despite—or through, or around—pain. *My space to live in may be tiny but I can work with it. I am brilliant at it.*

I managed to enjoy myself after all, despite everything.

We woke up together the next morning. While he showered, I stayed in bed, enjoying how sore and spent and relaxed I felt. My hips were heavy and easy and open. *Why had I let so many years pass without having sex?* I looked around his tidy studio, bathed in sunlight. His bed had sheets on it the American way, not just a duvet. It smelled clean, though there were plenty of strange and alien things. Dumbbells. Framed photos of athletes on the walls. Sports magazines were piled near his bed. I leaned over the edge of the bed and grabbed the closest one. I couldn't help but admire the extremity of all the elements in the cover photo. The saturation of color and movement and the body depicted: a football player seen from the back, stretching, jumping, reaching for the ball over his head, one foot still on the ground and the other lifted. Under synthetic fabrics, his buttocks were tensely laboring to protect his spine, they were hard, fixed objects sharply jutting out above his flatter, wider muscular thighs underneath. His back broadened dramatically up towards his sensationally expansive shoulders where well-developed, tan, tattooed arms sprouted. He was mid-movement, mid-extension, mid-giving it all, grunting, sweating, working. My shoulders would most likely be at his belly button level; his right arm stronger than my entire body.

Imagine living in such a big, utilitarian body; like a car, or a tree, or a bull—a body that could be spent as if strength, youth, and health are inexhaustible resources.

Since that first encounter, I sometimes notice glimpses of Nick's adolescence, the desensitization of his body when it was young and tender, the attempts at turning off feeling. *Run it off. Are you going to cry?* Violence as an ingredient, doled out with resolve for a specific effect. An attempt to clip the little thread that feels pain and vulnerability to keep it going endlessly without all the inconvenient parts. It's possible to squash natural feelings for a very long time. Maybe healthy, male bodies can do it forever, until they die from prostate cancer because they never saw a doctor.

Platter lift: a lift in which the man raises his partner overhead, with his hands resting on her hips. She is horizontal to the ice, facing the back of the man, in a platter position.

I catch my sister Ingrid on Skype. While it's evening for me, it's 3 a.m. for her. Her youngest is with her too, my adorable niece Solveig, who is a round and happy four-month-old baby. She can already recognize my face on the screen, and responds when I smile and imitate her noises. I long to hold her warm smallness in my arms. Ingrid and I have discovered that this is the best time to talk privately and comfortably, when she's up in the middle of the night with the baby, while my brother-in-law and nephew are asleep and Nick is out. She looks tired. Her breasts are large and full under her pajamas top, the wool inlays that would normally go in the nursing bra are now held in place by the thin fabric. Her hair is messy from sleep, her curls are gone ever since she had her first child. When Solveig is quiet and nursing, I tell Ingrid that I'm going to stop the injections that keep me in artificial menopause. "I want to try to get pregnant," I say.

Ingrid frowns. "I didn't even know you *could* go off that medication."

"Well, it is kind of risky..."

Solveig fusses in her arms and the sound makes the speakers blare. I raise my voice and keep talking though I'm not sure she can hear me.

"The endometriosis could flare up again and make the pain worse. But it's really not great to be on the medication for long either. It says in the leaflet that comes with the injections that you should never take it for more than six months, and I've been on it for three years! I told one of my doctors here how long I've been on it, and he was like 'Are you out of your mind?' Those exact words."

I pick up a pen from my desk and start clicking it.

"That doesn't sound too good!"

She sighs and looks away from the screen.

"Well, none of it sounds too good, really, when you look at it."

How does she get to tell me it doesn't sound good? The doctor also made sure to inform me that I have to be prepared for worse pain during a potential pregnancy, too. Whereas one of the most famous experts on endometriosis in New York city told me he could fix everything in an operation only *he* was skilled enough to do, which would pay him the equivalent of a yearly Norwegian salary. To prove that the operation was necessary, he conducted an examination so painful that I felt it for days afterwards. I surrender to a moment of hopelessness and sigh. Then I stop. I'm not going to give in to her naysaying. I straighten my spine.

"But it could turn out okay, still, you know? If I can get pregnant, that could have a positive effect on my pain. I mean, I'm going to have an MRI first to make sure my kidneys aren't in danger from the endometriosis. Apparently, some women lose their kidneys."

"Yay." My sister gives me a weak half-smile.

I'm hypersensitive to any indication that she's sick of my bad news. *I should be allowed to relate the basic facts of my life—even if that means MRIs instead of diapers and school runs—without that somehow being beyond the pale.* Anyway, I want this to be good news, and I want my fucking good news acknowledged when I have it. God knows it will turn around sooner or later.

"But Ingrid, this is good. I've decided to try to do this. Who knows, it might be fine."

"Well, congratulations. Good luck."

I can tell there's something she's not saying. She looks down at the baby's face.

"What?"

"I don't know. Are you sure about this? It's not easy. I mean, sometimes I would kill to be free and unencumbered in New York City."

Ingrid rubs her forehead. There are toys scattered around the living room behind her and several glasses and mugs on the table in front of the computer.

"I know it's not easy," I say.

Suddenly her vulnerability tips towards something almost angry.

"And, honestly, don't you want to come home to have a baby? Not only to have us close by to help out—and believe me you're going to need help—but I have ten months of fully paid maternity leave. I mean, that's a lot of money!"

This again.

"It's not easy for Nick to transfer to a country where he doesn't speak the language."

"Everyone here speaks English! Surely, he can design software here, too. And he could learn Norwegian."

The truth of it is that neither Nick nor I want to be in Norway, but I can't tell her that.

"Anyhow, I lost those benefits the moment I started work here. I think I'd have to work three years in Norway to earn the right to take maternity leave back. But, you know what, I have decent health insurance, you don't have to worry."

"Why did you start working in the US, then? Honestly, Laura!"

She sounds close to tears. She pushes her glasses up her nose, but before I can respond, Solveig squalls and Ingrid focuses all her attention on her. The conversation ends a short while after that.

Women with their babies, those eyes from inside the bubble. I'm on the outside. I can't argue that it's a rational choice exactly. It's part of the larger negotiation of safety versus risking big. Of staying in Norway versus going to New York. Of trying to get pregnant rather than giving in to the thought of everything that could go wrong. Knowing the dangers of your situation does not necessarily protect you. You can't be completely safe and get something out of life at the same time.

The best you can hope is to manage to be present enough and have some delicious moments on the way, a few things you can take with you when you cut your losses and escape into the wilderness. I've probably been influenced by my exile among Americans, by their ability to accept and even embrace the forces that shape their lives. When I first arrived in New York, I was mystified by the fact that there were so many more young people limping and using crutches on the streets in Harlem than in I'd ever seen in Norway. It's not as if these New Yorkers had chosen insufficient treatment of God-knows-what injuries and problems to live "more real" lives. Of course, they had no choice. Of course, it was a horror. But there was something in the way that situation was read from the safety of Norway that robbed these individuals with disabilities of some integrity, authority, some presence. Perhaps it was that American belief that they were, indeed, living in the best country in the world. All things considered, who am I to say those individuals lose rather than gain from that trust?

In the US, I feel like one person in an enormous world, whereas in Norway, I often felt like that one person in the room who, for some reason, drew more bad luck from the universe than the rest. It turns out that the rest of the world is more like me than it's like Norway. I'm more at home around people whose lives seem as hopeless and disrupted as mine does. My long list of allergies, which made me a freak growing up in the 1980s and '90s, barely raises an eyebrow in New York City. In general, American stories—from TV and books to snippets of conversations on the street—are bruised with terrible misfortune, and the people afflicted struggle in solitude, not only because of shame, but because they see some strength and honor in it, too. There are songs and expressions to stiffen your spine and there are ways for others to recognize your struggle. This country is such a confounding mixture of interdependence and freakish isolation, progressiveness and backwards thinking, charity and cruelty. There is no way to translate this into something my old country can understand. It's easier for them to see clichés and caricatures, to use "American" as a put down all on its own, like my mother still does.

There's something helpful to me about how New Yorkers aren't ashamed to ask for what they want. They aren't afraid people will think they're being difficult or trying to set themselves apart. Sure, good manners are expected, but New Yorkers don't hesitate to let their irritation show if they are treated badly. There's an emphasis on "the customer", which applies to so many more situations here than at home, whether it comes to seeing doctors or to tipping in restaurants. Being a New Yorker means being a person who has the right to make choices. It doesn't matter if I desperately need it or I just want it—I have the right to it. I can go somewhere else if I'm not satisfied. Taking up space and not giving a shit what anyone else thinks is a given here. You get more respect for being someone who makes demands, rather than being compliant. The distinction between worthy and unworthy needs that I grew up with is irrelevant. In this city, there's no question that I'm lucky compared to others with similar health issues. I'm independent—I make money, I have my education, and no one has to approve.

Perhaps it is simply a relief to be a person of privilege in New York, rather than a person who lacks privilege by comparison in Norway. More than once, I've had to contextualize my upbringing here—even though my father was a doctor, we didn't have a lot of money when I was growing up. In Norway, I was regular in every way—except I was sick. It's strange to feel safer here—but despite what you'd expect, the Norwegian safety net can make it feel necessary to be liked by people. Whatever you do is everyone's business. Everyone is reasonable, yet is aware of each other at all times, like siblings competing for a parent's attention. The downside to the many, many upsides.

When I left, there was some primal need for privacy twisting in me—to have no one watching me, to be left alone, to be able to do whatever I wanted and not have everything about me be rational and make sense. I felt like the fact of the loss of my health was acknowledged, but every response to the loss should be logical and it should be possible to explain myself at any moment. I wanted to rip loose instead, never clarify a single thing. I wanted blank space on my map.

It is extraordinary that a city could be so new that it could be based on ideas everyone agreed on, instead of growing randomly out of the ground like stalagmites, never to be changed, unless by fires or Haussmanns . Anyone who can count can find their way around New York City—and predict how long it will take to get there.

When my Norwegian family and friends visit New York, with their staring, clear eyes, they are so much rougher than Americans when they talk and not only because they're speaking a second language. They are always ready for a serious conversation about politics or morality. Making awkward faux pas in their eagerness to have opinions about things, using outdated vocabulary about race, but so excited to embrace New York, too.

My usual nightmare is back: *I'm in the ER in need of urgent surgery, in a state of pain and dread—hideous, unbearable defenselessness. The doctors and nurses keep misunderstanding me and making mistakes, they come and go and leave medical supplies lying around, and there is noisy chaos outside the room that distracts them from giving me proper care. I keep trying to get their attention, to get someone to help me. Nothing works. I'm stripped of any power. I'm imprisoned in my terrible body. I can't leave. Kjetil is there, as a little window I turn to in despair, his kind eyes looking at me helplessly. I always wake up without anyone having come to my aid.*

We live only in moments, one after the other. But there are days when the past is just too present. The horror isn't moment-shaped, it's a heavy mountainous gel, a frozen unmovable blob in which nothing can be changed. This moment, which forms a string of brand-new *this moment*s, becomes a forgotten sack of junk in the attic. I've had vivid nightmares since I was a child, but since my surgeries, they too have become a chronic illness of sorts. Maybe it's the hormonal changes from all the medications I've been on these past three years—or maybe it is PTSD. I suspect my days would be entirely different if I had Nick's deep, untroubled sleep, and never remembered a single thing my mind gets up to at night. My mind is like all the other parts of me—inflamed, hypersensitive, sore and scarred, working patchily, too much of some things and too little of others, the wrong tissue in the wrong place, reacting in the wrong way.

Though I've been increasingly healthy these past few years, both the pain and the nightmares remain. It feels like walking into a freezer, or rounding a corner to stumble upon a pile of dead bodies—suddenly finding myself in a state of complete and utter horror next to things that have already happened, that are completely unmovable. Those hospital nightmares leave me in the same state of nauseous terror all day afterwards. I try my best not to think about this extreme, repetitious panic.

After my conversation with Ingrid comes a night of nightmares, which always means waking up to a pain day. The pain is a half fallen-down wall of rocks around me, separating me from everything else. The degree of pain varies, but it always occupies a certain percentage of my life, whether a good month or a bad one.

I can tell I'm in trouble by listening to my breath. When I wake up from a queasy half-sleep, my breath is already a panicked animal high in my chest, a little voice saying in my native tongue, *Hvordan skal dette gå?* A lilting sentence heading right at the abyss, a sentence my mother would always utter with eyebrows raised and a small, smile-like grimace: *How on earth is this going to work itself out?* I strain to shut out every thought about everything that isn't right here, right now. I know from experience that everything in life feels completely impossible on a day like this. The life I'm already living is way too much, not to mention any lofty plans of what I could possibly achieve.

I lean, push, bump up against the pain. I try to stretch myself and reach over it to talk to Nick and get things done, but it is there. It wraps around my abdomen and pelvis, all the way up to my ribs, unmovable and merciless, just stuck. It's the kind of very unpleasant intestinal sensation that would typically only last a second before there is movement. It feels like things are literally stuck, aren't passing through my intestines, though they are: thank God, after all these years, I function normally again, more or less. Could it be referred pain from my pelvis? Who can make sense of all of this, after all this time? Pain has its own logic. It's a wall with no door, there is no arguing with it, no getting around it, no solving it. Sometimes, I bump against it like a fly against a windowpane for weeks at a time.

"Every single person arrives in the world like this," my friend Tatiana says. "There's no group of slightly less special people that came by freight train or elevator instead, you know?"

In the afternoon, Tatiana and I are in Riverside Park, discussing pregnancy. Tatiana is a good friend from school, who now works for a magazine. Her makeup is perfect, with expert cat eye flicks.

"I mean, giving birth, then the sheer amount of work of taking care of a baby…Are you sure?"

I smile at her. "I want to try, at least. I want to meet that little person."

People bustle around us. It's a hot day in June and I'm dizzy. I wish I'd brought a hat. The only free bench we could find is in the sun and I feel the sweat soak through my vintage sundress under my thighs. It has a Peter Pan collar and a high waist that accommodates my swollen, painful stomach. I'm not sure why I told her. I guess I want to conjure something good by letting a friend know that I'm going to try to get pregnant, but I'm too tired to defend myself when she offers up the reasons that I probably shouldn't. I try to make an active choice to focus on the soothing parts of the Tatiana experience rather than the points where we can't connect.

Maybe people aren't as mystified by pregnancy in Norway, or Texas, or someplace with spacious living rooms where having babies is what people do and everyone knows how. In contrast, my NYC-tribe of thin, tense over-thinkers aren't cool about this stuff at all. They flare up into alienation intertwined with tenderness and worry. One friend looked like she was going to faint when I told her about how, right before my sister gave birth, I could see the imprint of an actual little foot kicking against the tight skin of her stomach below her ribs.

"What about your health?"

Tatiana's long, curly black hair glints in the sun; she doesn't seem affected by the heat. I admire for a second how her olive skin glows in the heat. She eats too little and drinks too much, yet she's bursting with health. I close my eyes for a minute against the sun. Sometimes it feels like nobody can hear me when I talk. Nobody sees me if I don't spell out what the issues are in the most pedagogical way possible, and even then, most of what I'm saying gets lost in translation somewhere.

"We'll see. There'll probably be unpleasantness of some kind. There's definitely a risk. But I'm used to operating with bodily limitations, and all my doctors gave me the green light."

Granted, when I asked how pregnancy was likely to affect my severe endometriosis, which had caused adhesions all over my pelvis and abdomen and required surgery on my colon, one of my doctors (supposedly a specialist in this field), said: "I'll certainly be interested to find out."

The older we get, the more aware we are of what can go wrong. But we get more resilient, too—or so I hope. Yes, life is short and brutal and misfortune awaits around every corner—so we have to honor the moments untouched by cruelty and ugliness, some little part of ourselves that isn't hurt or at least can be healed. The ability to imagine something whole, beautiful and good. The camera zooms out from me, out of the bright, noisy moment where people move around us in the hot sunshine—up and out to include the grid of the enormous city, then further out to the edge of the continent, between oceans and mountain ranges, and even further out to the whole planet, surrounded by the cold, dark quiet of space. There, I can draw a calm breath. *All that being in place, what can we do?*

Other women do it all the time. Walk around with that stomach sticking out into the world showing everyone your outrageous vulnerability. What a ridiculous chance you're taking. Risking what health you have and assuming that there'll be a future, that there will be years ahead. As if all that was *given*—to *you*. Daring to assume that your life and your body can stretch to hold the weight of another human being.

I want to try.

I can try to own this choice while it's mine and not blame myself for my moment of hope if it all shatters. I've been taking my calcium pills and eating my kale. I try to shut the door on everything that can go wrong. Whenever people start talking about it, I will silence them with a look and a smile. *Whatever you've got there, keep it to yourself.*

Instead, I will keep repeating a few phrases to myself:

The tendency of human beings is to heal. I have the ability and power to make this decision. There is risk, but there is hope, too. There is loss, but there is beauty, too.

Because of my health issues, the window for getting pregnant is closing. If I want this life, I'd better try now. I want a life that resembles a regular life even if it isn't, even if no life is regular, even if no one gets everything they want and nothing is like it is on TV. I want a child.

As Tatiana leaves and I begin to make my way home, though, I feel how exhausted I am. The pain is there; it's been there the whole time. I've dosed the painkillers restrictively because the tiredness, nausea, and wooziness that accompanies them is so inconvenient. At some point, it becomes more difficult to change the plan than follow through, even if the plan is clearly too much for me. I take the painkillers now, knowing they will have a hard time capping the pain after so many hours, if they ever could have.

I'm too far away from any train station. I started my way home too late and I should have gotten a cab right away, but now I've already walked all these blocks and I'd have to walk several avenues to find a cab anyway. I sit down in the little park behind the statue of Jeanne d'Arc. There's no one else around. I flood with despair, which is as fresh as it's always been, despite mindfulness and meditation, therapists, surgery, drugs, and years. The nature of the despair hasn't changed in any decisive way.

It will never go away. I can't live with this. Even if it goes away later I can't stand it happening now.

I'm so sad, and so scared I can't even begin to know how to be okay with feeling it.

I can scarcely get through the days as it is, and there is no room, no margin to work with—nothing.

The thought of risking the health I have to try to get pregnant, risking getting worse, spending more time than this—or even *all the time from now on*—inside this pain spreads a chill through my chest. It's simply out of the question.

I guess I could do it by just doing it and ignoring my own objections. I could do all the planning on good days, and on the bad days, I could force myself to follow through, like when I was a child. It would be horrible perhaps, but not actually difficult for me to achieve. I can turn to stone and do anything I need to. It's not even a loud protest within me: it's something speechless and powerless that objects, a silent and tiny animal. There's no doubt as to what it wants, those small eyes on me. It's just a question of whether I honor it—or not.

The trees shield the little park from view and I am still alone. Dappled sunlight warming the cobblestones. I'm on the stone bench and see an older Black man walking towards me. He is wearing tinted eye-glasses and a military-print fishing hat pulled down around his face despite the heat. He's tied the leash of his dog around his very small waist, along with a fanny pack, and a worn plastic bag. *Shit, what's this?* He looks like he wants something from me. Instinctively, I plant my feet on the ground so I'll be able to leave if I need to.

"Excuse me," he says as he approaches, and I see that his face has been badly burned, probably a long time ago. "I'm deaf. Could you help me?"

He sits down on the stone bench next to me. I notice tears running down his mottled cheeks. His bottom lip is burned, too, and has been fashioned from other skin. His whole narrow face, even his very small nose, is made up of shiny scar tissue. *This is a man who has been fully drenched in pain, like a medieval saint.*

"We need her medication, I need to call, but I can't hear. I have a phone."

He gestures to his ears and I see that he's holding an actual ear in his hand, a brown silicone ear, lifeless yet completely lifelike. I try my best to choke back the horror I feel.

"Miss, could you call?"

He holds out his phone, an old model, already open to a listing for ASPCA in his contacts. I'm startled enough to take the phone from him.

"What do you need?"

I realize he must be reading my lips. His speech is perfect.

"We're all out of Maggie's pills. They sent my check to the old address 'cause I just moved and I went down there but they'd sent it back. They said it'll take a week to get to me. When I woke up I saw she'd been up running around last night and she'd been sick and I was there sleeping and I couldn't even hear her!"

His voice cracks and fresh tears start rolling down his face from underneath his tinted glasses. I might cry myself. The dog is clearly old and not in great shape—a big, golden cocker spaniel who lies on her side at his feet and turns around to look at me with round, dark eyes that have a bit of crust around them. Unlike her slight owner, the dog is portly. The man keeps up his tearful monologue, but I can't quite follow it. His crying sounds innocent, like a very young person's.

"Can you ask them if they can give out emergency medicine? It's twenty-two dollars. I went to the vet, but they wouldn't even give us a few pills to tide us over."

I press "talk" on his phone, even though I'm not sure what to ask for. It rings and rings.

Meanwhile, he digs around in his fanny pack and takes out an ID card that says "John Davis" under a New York benefits logo and lays it flat on the bench, along with a small orange box of pills, the name and type of medication worn away. There's also a pink Post-it where he's written in tidy cursive:

"Please call the ASPCA and ask if they can help get medication to Maggie: $22. I moved and my social security check was sent to the wrong address. Thank you, God bless, John."

I finally have a grasp of the situation. The complete finiteness of money when there simply isn't any—while other resources, like efforts to make yourself be liked and understood, can stretch endlessly. He has to rely on strangers for this last-resort phone call, most of whom would surely take one look and not even stop to hear him out—like I probably would have done on a normal day.

His burned face, his shabby clothes and all his plastic bags, his hunched posture, would all be read as reasons to back away—even if he kept his prosthetic ears on . No amount of planning perfectly polished words and gestures to combine with a disarming smile can solve people taking one look and reading you as dangerous. And yet he doesn't give up, because he can't save the dog himself. He must need his delayed check for other things, too, besides his dog's medication. The man is still crying. I find a Kleenex pack in my purse with one tissue left and I'm glad to have that to offer him.

I hang up the call after about fifteen rings.

"Maybe they're on a lunch break? I'll try again in a few minutes."

"Yeah. It's hard to get to them in the big city. Everything is harder here. The social security check takes so long and I, I only got these in March! I got burned…the system is real slow."

"You got burned in March?" I ask, horrified.

"No, no, I got *these* in March. I waited thirty years for them." He pops off his prostheses and shows them to me again. Perfect and useless silicone ears. Is that really the only help they have given him, prostheses to make him look more normal? Why not a video sign interpretation service? Here is this man, living in one of the most advanced and diverse cities on earth, without an ally in sight.

"Can I pet your dog?" I ask.

"Of course."

Maggie turns around and looks at me as I bend down and tentatively pet her back. Her fur is silky for such a scruffy-looking dog.

"So soft," I say before remembering that I have to turn my face to him for him to understand. I do, and repeat what I said.

"Yeah, softly like that," he says, thinking I'm reassuring him that I'm treating this old dog, his treasure, with care. He's still leaking tears.

I have cash in my purse. I can easily make this day less torturous for both him and the dog. "Can I give you the money?" I ask awkwardly. I don't want it to seem like he's asking me for it but the dog is clearly sick, and the man is in anguish. He must realize he will be without the dog soon, no matter what he does. His look is of intense relief, not offense, so I pull the cash and put it on the bench between us by the Post-it note, in an attempt to make it less awkward.

"Thank you so much! Oh, thank you! Now that vet can't say anything, he's getting paid in cash! Oh, thank you! I live close by—I could text you next week to pay you back, if you want to give me your number?"

His whole demeanor is changed by relief, his shoulders visibly relaxing, and his energy has returned.

"Please, it's okay," I say. "I can afford it this week." I'm immediately ashamed for the qualifier. I could afford it any week, when it truly comes down to it. Even now, I'm protecting myself from further involvement. Any other day I probably would have instinctively given anyone with worn plastic bags tied onto their person a wide berth , but I feel a pang when he shakes my hand and stands up. Giving him the money also means our conversation is over and that he'll take his bubble of loneliness and suffering with him.

"Good luck!" I blurt, but his back is turned already, his eyes on the dog.

I watch him go and the moment he's out of view, I realize I may as well allow the tears to come. After fighting them for a second, they arrive with gasps and actual sobs, like a little kid's. I cry with abandon. Every single human needs help from other people. But the opportunity to lean on someone isn't given to everyone. Sometimes there's only an absence like the open sky instead. A terrible loneliness glimpsed late at night when you are the only sober person in a room, catching the tired unhappiness pooling on a friend's face in between the animations of conversation.

A Latino couple strolls past me and takes a seat further down. The man is wearing a police uniform. I sense their presence and don't look up for a while, unable and unwilling to stop crying and be talked to, even by someone kind. Sometimes I can't stand always being surrounded by people in the city.

When I eventually look up, I see that they're kissing, slowly and intensely. The man's face is soft with tenderness, his eyes closed. The woman's hands are paused midair in her lap in the middle of unwrapping their take-out.

I get home, finally. I drop my things in the hallway and wash my hands before I flop down on the couch next to Nick. He stretches his neck and kisses my hair. He smells a little funky and is working on something on his computer. I lean on his shoulder, even though we are both sweaty. He doesn't speak for a while, then looks up and tenderly says: "Darling, you look like shit."

I laugh in spite of myself and then I cry a little more. He puts his arms around me and I close my eyes and put my cheek against his neck. I'm comforted, and I wonder if he knows anything about what's going on with me, and whether it matters.

Afterwards, I have a decent nap and I feel a bit better. Over dinner, as my blood sugar stabilizes, I listen to Nick explain what he's been working on and I feel hope light up again in my chest. It just happens. I can try. *I'll try.* I regard myself with surprise. *So that's what you want? You are willing to sacrifice and take risks for a child, after all?*

Looks like it.

There is an inviolable expanse of blue sky inside me: the sky of a spring evening, running around and playing and laughing with my big sister and the older kids on our street, sneakers pounding the dry, pale Norwegian tarmac with the small, rounded stones in it, ankles and feet unused to the sensations and freedom of *småsko* after endless months of winter boots. *Leke i gaten.* I'm the youngest in the bunch, but allowed to play with them if I run fast and don't whine. We hide and seek in the gardens and chase each other in the street, the cool clean air. Our fingers chilly beneath the sleeves of the unfamiliar lightness of a denim spring jacket. Screams and laughter echo. The fun doesn't end because the light just *stays* and the bright sky is like everything exciting and new and promising. The blue deepens, dusk stretches out, but the sky never yields to darkness.

PART 3

OBLIVION

2010

When things feel impossible during my first six months in New York, instead of repeating the mantra my therapist in Oslo suggested—Everything is all right, Laura, I furiously think: *I'll kill myself,* over and over and over until the situation passes. Then I try my best to forget it immediately, forget everything. When I'm writing, or when it's all too much, I sense an edge where it seems like I could dissolve and disappear and it's what I want.

I haven't talked to Kjetil in three days. My mother visited for a week and stocked my apartment with laundry detergent, groceries selected to make easy dinners, allergy food, and bedsheets brought from home. Now that she's gone, I lose myself in all the American things I have to sort out—banks, doctors, schoolwork, parties, not to mention cheerful, drunk conversations with students who are all on their best behavior, like me. Seeing people at school is good—is enough. Everyone is so nice and understands me, or so it seems, although I hardly share anything about myself. I bury myself in schoolwork and writing, which is what I came here to do. It feels good to focus on that even if it's all clearly too much and I'll never get everything done. I text Kjetil that I don't have time to talk during the small window of time in which our days overlap, between his work and bedtime, six hours ahead of me. I can't explain this to anyone. I don't exactly realize that I'm doing it. When we do talk, I fill our conversations with stressed-out monologues about everything I have to do and how impossible it is. It *is* almost impossible. I have to ration my energy. I need, I absolutely *need,* to manage my schoolwork. I'm not out of the woods by any count.

My father calls. At the end of the conversation he casually asks about Kjetil.

"He's still looking for work here."

"He's still coming? Has he had any leads?"

"Not really. It's very difficult to find work in New York. He needs an employer to sponsor his visa. It actually costs a lot of money."

"So, he's going to wait for you, huh?"

"We're hoping he can find a job…"

"But you think he's going to wait two years for you and hold down the fort, while you're on a different continent having the time of your life?" He no longer sounds casual. "After he took care of you this spring?"

"Well, that's his choice, isn't it? I'm not making him do anything. He encouraged me to go!"

"It's not easy for him, you know. It's not easy to take care of you. You should give that some thought. If you leave him alone like this, who knows what will happen?"

"But he's not taking care of me now! He doesn't have to worry about me anymore! Anyway, do you seriously not think any of this has crossed my mind?"

"I just think that you should be grateful for all he's done for you."

"I *am* grateful! You be fucking grateful!"

I hang up the call, breathing hard and burst into tears.

I can't tell him I can't stand the idea of keeping Kjetil or losing him. I can't stand to think of our old life—the apartment he calls me from and our plans, the future that used to exist, the future we dreamed of. My brain is overloaded. I can't think about what he's thinking or how he's feeling.

I miss him so badly it's like a wound that keeps bleeding. I have to close it somehow, or it will kill me. I can't have him here with me. I cannot, I *will not* go back.

When people let all their angriest, most scared, most hopeless stuff out, it doesn't sound like it does on TV: well-phrased, dignified, and attractively tragic. It's violent and awful, revolting even. If I were in his shoes, I would not be able to stand it. Not being able to fix it. Getting stuck with all the boring chores, along with being pinned to the wall to witness the worst possible shit you could imagine happening day after day and night after night. Tears and vomit and being woken up again and again by groaning. Hanging around the hospital bed sadly stroking your lover's forehead and holding their hand while all your own emotions store up and you can't talk to them because they're asleep, on morphine and struggling. They need you so badly. *How strong does love need to be to withstand the point where continuing means self-destruction?* Every direction you can move in is unforgivable.

There are those first three months or so when you are seeing someone new, and you only get the cream, and then you can just move on to the next one, right?

I can't even stand to think it. I have to let go.

Flying back sit spin changing the foot of landing: A spin involving a jump form a forward outside edge to a backward outside edge, landing in full back sit position.

It's not disastrous to not have enough; you can turn to strangers or friends, or even say, *"I'm sorry, I just can't manage, I need more."* The deadly thing is not to go without, but to pretend the crumb is enough—that it's natural for you to not be seen or to receive, that there is no loss, that you have no bigger plans anyway. To be so scared of losing that crumb that you can never say how hungry you are for more. To feel such shame about the need itself that exposing it for even a second is dangerous. To be so apologetic about how much trouble you are that you spend your life hiding and shutting up, being grateful you even get that morsel.

It's a question of poverty on some level, because if I lose a lot, I better hold on to what's left—otherwise, what the hell do I expect? How furious that idea makes me, even at Kjetil. *Why should I not want to rob him blind, rather than take his charity?* I'm not a helpless child, not anymore. There is a point where I am unwilling or unable to budge. Call it an inability to process my situation or whatever you want. *I don't want it.*

I never want to need anyone ever again. My life is limited. I can't take long, time-consuming detours anymore. I have to go straight there. I have to burn it all to the ground or I won't survive this. The destruction has to be so complete that it closes all windows to the past, until there's nothing left but a big burnt scar on the ground and smoke tearing through my lungs, my hands black with soot. Nothing to do but turn and walk away. Either survive without or not survive at all.

I have difficulty resting. Sleep is hot and shallow. My mind is never quiet, yet it feels like a scorched, empty landscape. Dull, nauseous pain trembles up through the arid ground and worries the air like a heat haze.

I don't have time to panic or doubt. Feverish, fuming thoughts make so much constant noise, I can almost ignore it. I work until a hot flash comes and then I stop and wait it out, eyes fixed somewhere beyond the horizon, the radio broadcast of fury turned up to a blaring volume washing over me with the heat. I hope people don't notice how much I blush and sweat. I've barely done either before in my life. I've prided myself on maintaining a certain level of dignity and control over my body no matter what, particularly over my appearance. For all the good that did me.

I've been some version of a pretty girl since my mid-teens. These are different times. I don't look remarkable. I just look old, miserable, bloated, defeated. Everything is difficult with this exhausted body, with this uncomfortable, swollen stomach. I alternate between feeling desperate to look how I used to and anger at being shut out from anything that's fun and young, between the desire to be invisible and grief at being invisible. I'm lonely, yet glad there's no one else's healthy sexuality to deal with anymore. The very last thing I need is someone trying to have sex with me, and having to put a happy face on that shit show. For the past six months, having intercourse has become something akin to a medical procedure—possible to carry through to its end, but not recreational. My body doesn't want to. It's as if I'm a virgin again, but much worse, because I'm no horny, slinky teenager with her life ahead of her. It's felt both gross and sad to go through with it and pretend it's enjoyable on a rare occasion. I couldn't see any alternative to pretending. Getting Kjetil off on his own would seem like the solution, but that doesn't feel like fun either. That would only highlight how nothing is how it used to be; how I'm not the way I'm supposed to be.

I hope he hasn't realized nothing is fun for me. I couldn't let every situation that curves towards a scene of weary tears just go there. There would be nothing else. I was a bad enough girlfriend already.

One class on Mondays, Wednesdays, and Fridays, two on Thursdays. I get through the days. I congratulate myself for looking like a regular-enough person, at least most of the time. During the second week of classes, I get called on while I'm staring into the air across the big table and I make a complete fool of myself, stuttering in staccato, babyish English. Two of the American students pounce on my helpless assessment of the piece we read and interrupt each other with mellifluous orations about how wrong I am. I sit there blushing, wishing I were dead. But the girl sitting next to me jokes with me about it after class and I feel better.

I try to always keep a couple of extra dinners in the apartment, in case of bad days. I take taxis when I get groceries. When I go out, I only drink ginger ale in a whiskey glass, so it's not obvious that I'm not drinking. I look forward to getting home so I can cry. The last three years' respite from facing things head-on alone is over.

Maybe I never really had it any other way. *Is it even possible for people to accompany each other to the darkest places?* It seems to me that the point where anything really helps me is much further down the line than the point where it starts to be too much for other people, or even hurt them. On a scale of impossibility, it's slightly less impossible to manage on my own. Loneliness and grief are a smaller price to pay than the hell of needing so horribly, so helplessly, and being let down, rejected. Kjetil always said that it didn't matter that it was difficult, because I was what he wanted. But I realize with some shock that despite the grief that chokes me, I can manage without him.

"Well, we're all terminal," says my therapist. "People with terminal cancer just may know how it will happen or have a more specific timeline than the rest of us. There's always the clear message that if you get better, then you have to reenter the responsible world again. But while you're sick, you're sort of allowed to do what you want, right?

"It's the words people use, too, heroism and war, 'You're gonna beat this thing! Keep fighting!' 'So and so lost the battle against cancer…'," she continues. "No one's going to hold it against you if you want to go climb mountains or swim with dolphins or do whatever you want with your life if you have terminal cancer.

"But, for some reason, people who get serious chronic illnesses don't get treated that way. Instead they have shame. They often feel they have failed somehow."

After starting the injections that keep me in menopause at twenty-nine, my life acquired an element of slapstick. I think I've read some comic strip on this theme. Some hot and bothered woman drawn with zig-zags of stress coming out of her head, a blushing face and a wailing mouth, eating chocolate and fanning herself. Fucking *hilarious.*

I try to remind myself that it's all about framing it right: *I'm lucky it isn't cancer, it's amazing compared to the alternatives, it's almost natural. Anything that stops the pain is worth it.* But the pain isn't even gone and furious tears keep returning at the most inappropriate times of the day, along with a desire to throw tantrums. It's absurd that what tips people from the ranks of adults over into the less cute ranks of being *old* also strips you of your ability to behave like a grown-up.

I think of my aunt Elsa, who's always been a model of dignified adult behavior for me. She recently turned fifty and is still leading a stylish life in London. She let her hair turn silver. She's never let on any trouble with hot flashes or anything else. Her health is impeccable, like her manners. I wonder how old she'll get before her bodily frailties start to resemble mine.

The first hot flash was nothing more than a little frisson, like blushing lightly all over. *Finally, something that isn't as bad as they say,* I actually dared to think. A few months later, I wake up glowing with heat and bathed in sweat every night. The generous heating in my apartment is now an unbearable annoyance. The entire world can, in a second, transform into a crowded sauna with no exit. A surge of heat starts on my back below my bra and spreads up the back of my neck and over my forehead. Then sweat breaks out all over my body. I've never sweated so much in my life. The hottest areas are the small of my back and the back of my neck, the hair on the back of my neck soaks right through.

I'm aware without being able to help it that my face is drawn, like when you put your fingers on a face made of clay and mess it up, pull at it just a little so its entire character is changed. I'm *aging*. A deep frown settles, and my eyes irrevocably start to belong on a sad face. Something people might snag on, look again, because I look awful, heartbroken. I used to see people like that, sometimes, and imagine they were going through a divorce, or their father, their mother or—God forbid—their child had died. People who couldn't muster up the energy to hide what was going on with them and conform their faces to what the world expected.

One day, during my first few weeks in New York, I sat across from a stylish middle-aged lady with sharp Louise Brooks hair on the subway. The toes of her lace-up boots were turned towards each other. Suddenly, her perfectly painted mouth opened like she was about to scream for her life. I braced myself, but it was just a yawn—just what a yawn looked like on someone for whom nothing was ever all right.

Clothes turn into a sudden terror. Even if I could undress in the middle of school or on the subway, I wouldn't be able to get them off fast enough. When the hot flashes happen, I want to tear at my throat. All these garments hemming me in, clasps and straps and hooks and zippers and buttons holding me down, choking me. My hair is in my face all the time, and this cut doesn't even look good. I have to angle my shoulder to keep my purse strap on it while carrying bags of heavy groceries on the subway—people never give up their seats—and not lose my gloves or hat in the freezing wind outside. It all becomes unbearable. So many parts of daily life are painful and annoying.

A sudden enormous anger at all of it slams into me with an intense desire to tear, kick, ruin, and break. People in my way, the paper bags containing heavy blue cabbage I bought to get some of those healthy whatevers that dark-colored vegetables have. Does cabbage even contain it? Or was that just the leafy stuff? Cabbage devoid of antioxidants, heavy, upsetting to the already upset stomach. *Why did I even buy the stupid thing!* Oh, for the love of *God*! I find myself thundering curses at inanimate objects that don't work, things that spill and fall, stinky staining oil from the expensive sardines I try to eat for my bone density's sake. Things dropped, broken and trailing behind me, stacks of clothes falling out of the closet when I try to get a box of papers down without bothering to get a chair to stand on. *Fuck you, fucking behave your fucking self you fucking goddamn piece of shit!* I have to invent new curses to fit all my anger, the indignity of it all, creating phrases I'm glad no one is there to witness. *Ratmonster fuckshit! Assbastardbloodycrapfuck!*

Estrogen pills limit the hot flashes and make me look prettier, but the pain worsens. I have to manage with just the fake estrogen that barely caps the hot flashes but hopefully still protects my bones enough. In the months following my first injections my eyes are less clear. I stare in horror at my hair which seems duller and thinner in the mirror. My lips less red. My skin less supple, but hairier. All the little flaws in my beauty are beginning to accumulate and I'm losing under this overwhelming attack from all angles. My crow's feet, which my old friend Marius once proclaimed charming. I saw them as charming when they were one element in the smooth, well-composed disk of my face. Not now. My slightly discolored teeth, the broken veins in my cheeks—what have I done to deserve them? They've certainly not come from excessive pleasure, from long nights partying, drinking, and smoking. I'm not attractive and I'm not okay but at least I'm alone and it's no one's business but mine. There's no one in New York City that knows any other version of me. They think I really look like this.

The idea of suicide is something I've never allowed myself until now, like it's a treat of some kind. Not even a thought—an image that flashes through my head, without any real emotion attached. *Folding my body through the open bottom half of my window.* The fall is so readily available. All I'd have to do is raise the screen. These thoughts have never been mine, and if they reared their heads, they were beaten down immediately. Unthinkable. But I'm so tired and so angry. I allow them to flow over me like cool, soothing water. The world is spinning out of control. I'm constantly holding down one thing only to turn and watch something else fall off the shelf and shatter, the eternal force that says all things are forever becoming more and more fucked up.

You have it, and suddenly it is gone, it's over. You should have used it better. The world shrinks and shrinks. You can't keep anything. Only the knowledge that you shouldn't have been worried, should've been happy while you could.

The gastrointestinal specialist is in his seventies and I can tell the whole integral health thing is a little new to him. His office is pleasant, with soft carpets and Native American sand paintings. My general practitioner, who referred me to him, sent him forty-six pages on me that are now up on his screen. It's some stuff from Norway and all the tests we did here. "So, you continue to improve," the doctor says.

He quotes what I said last time. I can't remember that I was worse. Or that I'm doing better now. But it's true. We've been testing new drugs, and this last one seems to be working. I'm sleeping a little better for one thing.

"Are you physically active?"

"I run sometimes and do some yoga. I try to do it twice a week, but—"

"You run?" He's clearly shocked.

"I try to."

Before I go, he stops me to say I'm doing a lot better than he expected.

"You're exercising, you're going to school, look at you," he says, beaming.

I walk out into the sunshine feeling my usual post-doctor fatigue. But I feel *happy,* too.

Third day on painkillers. I'm on my way to a specialist. Immobile on an orange plastic seat on the D train, I realize the walk to the station was too much and I'm completely drained. I don't think I can even stand up. I let my head fall back against the ad poster behind me and close my eyes, allow the train to rock me. So far, I've always managed to push myself just a little longer, as long as I need to go. By the time I arrive, I'll most likely make it up the stairs. But I probably shouldn't be running my life like this. I can't take it for granted. Everything crumbles.

On the way to the station I heard a nice melody from an open window. Spring. My head is churning, as usual, both worsened and comforted by the codeine.

Why do I draw the lightning out of the sky, while others have a safe, clear road for years and years? The absolute worst thing is to be someone else's inspirational story, where they see you and think: "Everything is okay as long as I don't have what you have." Why should I give a shit whether *you* make the most of your blessed cream cake life ?

Then again, there's always someone who is worse off than me. I can't wait for the trouble to pass. I have to take good times where they appear. As long as I can walk down the street and listen to music, make eye contact with people, wear my own clothes, as long as everyone is alive and healthy and I'm a certain measure of okay, not in *too much* pain and not deteriorating with a fixed end date. So, shut up and feel lucky, damn it. Act immediately to protect feelings of happiness, peace, and calm when they appear. Knock on wood.

Avoiding those bitter thoughts could be as easy as the express train gliding past that station without stopping. Don't go there. But already it's too much. It's too much before I even begin.

Take the first doses of medicine and supplements with breakfast, spreading the tablets out through the meal with the right amount of water to prevent nausea. Wash my face carefully. Put cream on my scars to fade them. Plan how long my nap should be. Open the window. Wipe down the table. Take breaks and stretch to prevent tendonitis from bad posture. Do some exercises to improve my posture. Plan doctor visits in-between schoolwork and classes, along with therapist appointments, the chiropractor, and the acupuncturist. Send insurance paperwork. Get to the pharmacy. Run in the sunshine to prevent pain and inflammation and to build strength and bone density. Listen to mindfulness meditation recordings. Cook food for later to prevent getting too hungry and to make sure to eat only balanced and gentle meals. Kale, vegetables, quinoa, fatty fish. Sweep the floor. Write. Rest.

PART 4

NEVER LET ME GO

2010

We spend the first two days of our vacation on the beach, swimming in the clear water—my father, Ingrid, my brother-in-law, their son and me. Kjetil is at home, working. He doesn't seem to have a lot of fun these days. When we talk on the phone in the evenings, he is always on the verge of falling asleep in front of the TV. *Is he relieved I'm away?* He can finally just eat takeaway food and get some rest after the horror of the past few months.

My nephew loves the surf. He hangs from my hand, his tiny soft hand clutching my fingers, kicking the water and jumping back towards my legs, squealing joyfully when the waves come back. He's so small and light that he doesn't wear me out too quickly. He has a round little belly, thin arms and legs and a blue sun hat, and when he laughs it's one of the few things that make me laugh too.

I'm "out of the woods for now", according to my doctor, and I'm supposed to be healing by the day. I'm still tired all of the time and my thoughts are weirdly slow. Sounds are too loud. All day long, my head buzzes like a broken bulb from the nightmares about the hospital I still have every night. That alone seems to take 50 percent of my capacity. They're not so much dreams as time travel. I'm back there, strapped in and spread-eagled on the table in a half-lit room with the nurses busy around me, getting the needles and my arms ready for the anesthesia. I feel the sterile green cotton socks tighten stiffly around my toes; I feel the padded stirrups under my knees and the elastic of the surgical hat around my forehead. I hear my thin, desperate voice telling them about my mother, who is a nurse too, just to get them to talk to me. I smell the disinfectant they will use on my skin. The light is in my eyes.

I wake up in horror—sweating, mid-hot flash, nauseous, and exhausted. I can't shake the feeling through the day, the sensation of surgical socks constricts my toes even when I run them through the sand, hard. I can't get out of my body, where the memories echo as if I need to learn something vital from them. They are more real than the present and I don't have the words or the occasion to explain it to anyone. Everyday conversations are inadequate; my illness is already old news to my family. We've worn away the most necessary things to talk about and now most conversations are about my nephew and things we see and eat. I mention that I have nightmares. They know I had surgery, but it was two months ago, so why should we talk about it now? We hardly mention my upcoming move to New York either, which is supposed to take place in a few months. Talking about it might tempt fate. Besides, I wonder if they think I'm delusional to still believe it can happen. There are too many unanswered questions and I overload immediately when I try to think about it. I barely have the energy to carry my own stuff during the short walk to the beach.

In the evenings, after my sister and her family are in bed, my father and I sit on the balcony and look at the sea. I try to keep up with my family, smile, be cheerful—especially with my nephew—but there's a thick veil over everything. For the first time since I was fourteen, men don't look at me at all on the beach. My stomach is swollen, my posture terrible. My eyes peer out unhappily from my puffy face. I can't help thinking of the person I was when I was here, just a year ago. The person I was then looked a lot better in this very same bikini. She wasn't startled by the waves and she was making plans.

The fact that I can't find a bathroom quickly enough on the beach is constantly on my mind. I stay behind, by the kidney-shaped pool. There's no one around and it feels good to be alone. I cover all my scars in thick layers of sunblock before meandering around to smell all the various roses that bloom abundantly around the patio. Then I lie down gingerly on the row of brown stone tiles that line the edge of the pool. The warm, slightly rough stone surface feels good against my back and I soak up warmth from below and from the sun above. The sky is a deep, clear blue. An insect of some kind hums. A dog barks in the distance. When I blink my eyes, I glimpse only light and fresh, pastel colors. I trail one hand through the cool water while the other rests on the warm stones, and I suddenly feel something give a little, feel myself start to relax. Only then do I realize I haven't done so in a very, very long time.

I'm back in Bergen to see my family and sort things out for my move to New York. Kjetil is at home in Oslo, working, as always. My mother accompanies me to get a nurse at a public vaccination clinic to sign the papers for the American university. The clinic's records aren't complete, since I received some of the vaccines at the hospital under special supervision due to my hyper-allergy to the eggs they were made with.

My mother is absolutely positive I had the injections, even though they're not in the system.

The nurse looks up from her files and says: "You were six, don't you think you'd remember if you had to go to the hospital?"

My mother and I exchange looks.

As we get back in my mother's car, I'm exhausted. The pain is there; I realize it's been there for hours.

"What does Kjetil think about you taking off like this, by the way, when he still hasn't found a job there?" my mother says, eyeing me as she turns on the ignition. "You have to know it's not easy for him."

Here we go.

"I don't want to talk about this," I respond through gritted teeth.

I take the new light rail to the center of Bergen to go see some friends. The light rail has recently started running after the building process was stalled for years, and I'm uncontrollably irritated with the people sitting around me for how excited they are about it, their stupid, happy exclamations. I stuff headphones in my ears and turn up the music as a hot flash comes on, thinking *Fuck this.* I hate everyone and everything. Nothing helps. *I need to sleep for a year. I need to be left alone.* I can barely stand talking to my friends, which is supposed to be fun. I want people to be shaken by what I tell them, but either they don't give a shit or they always saw my life ending up like this: miserable. When they go on talking about themselves as if nothing happened, as if we're exchanging news from a regular six-month period in our lives, as if everything is on track, I feel like I might scream.

I'm not okay. I'm not okay. I'm not okay.

My mother says her friend who had a mastectomy was told it would take a year before she got used to her new body. I think to myself, *I'll kill myself if anything more happens.* But then it does.

Jumps: Jumps are really spins in the air.

It's two weeks before I'm supposed to leave for New York and from the moment I open my eyes in the morning I have a feeling that something will go wrong. I lie there for a minute looking at the white ceiling in the dim bedroom that we never manage to de-clutter completely, trying to find the energy to get up anyway. I try to ignore these mornings. I have them so often. It's extra terrible when something happens on a day like this, as if someone is proving a point to me.

I have a doctor's appointment and end up spending all my time with her talking about the worsened abdominal pain I've been having for a few days, instead of the paperwork I came for. I've been coming here at least once a week for months doing exactly that—postponing the actual issue for a more urgent problem and scheduling a new appointment on the way out.

Last night, Kjetil and I looked up my new address in New York on Google Earth, cuddling on the corduroy couch in our living room and writing lists of what to pack. It was a pleasant little thing in the middle of an enormous to-do list I'm struggling with. I'm running on nothing but nervous energy. It still feels unlikely that I will actually leave Norway and go to New York, but the ticket is paid for and every day that goes by, the rest of the world takes my plan more seriously.

Kjetil keeps reassuring me that I can do it. When I transferred the tuition money (all my savings plus new, staggering student loans), I had to keep repeating to myself, *I can get it refunded.* The contrast between my life at the moment and the plan I worked out before I got sick—leaving everything to get a degree that would have intimidated even a regular person—makes the whole thing seem ridiculous. It also means giving up the social security benefits I'm living off of at the moment. But I can't let the chance pass me by without at least trying. There is no other plan.

Anyhow, if it goes to hell I won't be any worse off. People around me are eager to have a reason to be happy for me. They keep exclaiming how great it is that I'm going. It means leaving behind Kjetil, who has his job in Oslo. Of course, he will be joining me later—if there ever is a later. He's been trying to find work in New York every possible way for months with no luck. We were piled on top of each other on the couch, gazing at the tree we think of as ours outside the window, and we wrote lists of what we were looking forward to doing in New York. *Shopping for clothes*, I wrote . He put down *MoMA. Coney Island. Drinking beer on a fire escape.*

My doctor, a short-haired young woman, has me lie down on the examination table in her bright office to examine my painful and sore stomach. I look mostly at the ceiling while she looks at my impassive face, trying to gain information from it, pressing the palm of her hand into my skin and tapping the back of her hand with her fingers. Hard pressure, then release, asking again and again what hurts more, while I do my best to answer accurately. Lately, I at least have the attention of my doctors. But my face doesn't reflect how I feel.

The second surgery has, to the best possible degree, corrected the causes of my pain, and its nature has been shifting slowly. The wounds on the outside of my stomach have healed, but the pain is still here. The digestion stops, starts, cramps, hurts. One afternoon it's a little better, and then it's just as bad for weeks, as if it will never lessen at all. It's anyone's guess whether it ever will, or whether the damage is too extensive. My head is full of images of rocks and frozen, muddy gravel—jagged, dirty, unmovable things. Surgery causes new scarring and adhesions even when the purpose of the surgery is to remove the problematic tissue. The body can take a lot of beatings, but there is always a price to pay. Surgery is an exhaustible resource for my condition. Beyond that, there are the hormonal mind and body-altering injections that I'll stay on indefinitely, with lists of serious and bizarre side effects the length of my arm. There are other drugs to balance them with dangerous side effects of their own. It's crystal clear to me that no one wants to hear about it, but I will never finish needing to tell how much it hurt, how much it hurts, how bad it is. I'm always looking for a scale to measure it by, some way to pierce the thick skin that separates me from other people, to make them understand.

My doctor tells me this new pain isn't a new or acute problem. Just a variation in the daily pain, which might go away on its own. When you have pain for a long time, your body becomes more and more skilled at experiencing that pain. So much traffic transforms the neural pathways into highways. On the tram home though, I become certain beyond any doubt that it is something. I try to sit perfectly still, breathe shallowly, not cause any disturbance—a finely tuned balancing operation. There's either falling down into the chasm or staying on the line. I count down the stops, my breaths, and, when I finally get off the tram, the meters left in the short walk to my building, to the gate, down the hallway, the steps up the stairs—fifteen, fourteen, thirteen, twelve, eleven…Finally, I fit my key into the lock with shaking hands, barely make it through the door, drop my keys and tear at my jacket. I bring my bag with my phone to the bathroom just in case, shoes still on.

The stomach is the soft point of the human body. It has the largest number of nerves outside the brain and is sometimes called the second brain. Pain gets distorted and echoes around, making it hard to tell where it is coming from. 95 percent of the primary visceral nerve, the vagus, carries information from the gut to the brain and not the other way around. When the stomach is compromised, you feel like you're dying, even if it's nothing dangerous. When it finally stops, it feels like salvation. You vow to never take your health for granted again. It is no coincidence that lots of shamanistic rituals and planned transcendent experiences start with a good purging.

There is no wonderful relief once I finish throwing up. It's the first time I've vomited since I had the intestinal surgery a few months ago. There are only a few seconds of ease, then the pain starts up again. A steady crescendo. *Shit.*

The second woman I shared a room with at the hospital said it felt like a knife in her belly when her operating wounds got infected. She was so eager to get home and see her little blond grandson. *Where did I get that he was blond from?* I sit down on the floor carefully and slowly unlace my shoes. Then I grab a towel and walk slowly to the kitchen listing what I need to do in order of importance. Water first. A bucket. Rice cakes. Maybe if I put something in my stomach, it will settle a little. Afterwards, I make my way to the couch, spread the towel on it, and gingerly try to lie down.

My life as I once knew it, in which I could get fairly predictable results from what I did to my body, a life of exercise, parties and work, is completely gone. This version doesn't even remotely resemble the old one. I've been trying to wait the pain out, like a nine-month cold—unpleasant but not meaningful—but the darker moments, when I suspect that my old life isn't coming back, are becoming more frequent. I hold all the unthinkable truths about my body and life in my head, untouched, waiting for a time when it will be possible to look at them. They're heavy pool balls, rolling around and bumping into each other.

I just need one problem to be solved, or at least have its skin broken before I can deal with the rest. Instead, more and more weigh down on me. I just need one good day to sit down, put them on the table, and look at them separately, with a clear eye and solve each problem like a puzzle, maybe even find something that could help several at once. Something that won't make the digestive problems worse, that won't make me throw up, or feel dizzier or give me headaches, because all those symptoms are past capacity.

There must be something I can do, some sort of penitence, or level of enlightenment I can ascend to. I can give up ever eating anything tasty again, no problem, eating has already been a chore for nine months. I can exercise and take every kind of vitamin, mineral or supplement under the sun. I can do without working, without going out, drinking, even without friends. I can find some way to meditate the trouble away. If there are monks who can raise their temperatures and levitate through meditation, then I can find a way to manipulate this body and make it livable. If I spend three hours a day doing it, I could learn how, surely.

If only I didn't have to take quite so many painkillers, I could think a little straighter and find a way to live with it. If only I could sleep. If only I could have one doctor-free day. If only I didn't have to spend all my energy on dressing, showering, keeping food down, getting the minimum done. If I didn't have to get these injections that sit like an enormous wasp's sting under the skin, if I could at least take medications that didn't worsen each other's side effects, as if someone had worked it out like that on purpose. If only I could think clearly for five minutes.

Yet again, I text Kjetil to eat something on the way home so there aren't any food smells at home. When he comes home from work, he finds me in my pajamas, pacing the living room, clutching my stomach. It's an overcast day. I can't concentrate on reading. I can't watch TV; any conflict or unpleasantness onscreen makes me feel worse. We try to watch TV, but I can't focus and take to pacing again. I drink in small sips but the water feels like poison in my stomach. I shuffle into the bathroom and throw up again. I try to sleep a little and I ask Kjetil to massage my back. He takes all his cues from me and does everything I ask. He's used to seeing me like this, and seems to pause himself until the crisis passes. Is he holding his breath hoping all will go back to normal soon? At some point, like everything else, it'll have to be dealt with.

Throw jump: a move in which the man assists his partner into the air and she performs the necessary rotations and landing.

My sister pointedly asked: am I relying too heavily on Kjetil? He did the housework, administrative tasks, difficult phone conversations with strangers, reassurance, comforting, anything that requires bending over, walking, and carrying something for long. I'd even toned down our actual domestic life in the recounting, trying to make it funny, somehow, that he had to wait on me.

"Doesn't he get sick of you?"

That was her focus, that I should know that I was impinging on someone, that I really should consider reining this whole embarrassing thing in somehow, not the fact that I actually needed this much help. I felt my cheeks flush.

"Well. It's not like anyone else is helping me out."

My voice sounded breathless and cold. I could tell she was startled by my sudden shift. She looked away and changed the subject. I let her talk. The unsaid things kept echoing in the kitchen. I could hardly believe the distance between our realities. As if this were a situation in which reasonable adults could make choices based on what was a better alternative, not this post-apocalyptic wasteland in which I'm scrambling for my life. I couldn't even imagine surviving if Kjetil were any less supportive. What on earth did she suppose I could do differently? Even with the maximum restraint on my behalf, even with everything that he gives, my need is still always bigger. Kjetil can't save me from anything, even if he is the most generous partner I've ever had. It's yet another thing that doesn't add up.

I'm beginning to suspect we are going to have to do something about the state I'm in, but I'm in too much pain to consider it. It's easier to put the thought off, for just a little longer. Finally, I stand up and call my father, always my first go-to with medical issues.

He's clear; "Call an ambulance, immediately."

The two paramedics take the long straight boulevard up, up, up. I can see Oslo flatten out through the window in the back of the ambulance. I tell the paramedic who rides in the back with me that I'm supposed to move to America in two weeks.

"If this is an infection related to the surgery, they can sort that out pretty quickly. But it's probably just a virus. Two weeks is a long time! Don't worry." There's a rehearsed reassurance in his tone as he attempts to get one of my surgeons on the phone. I briefly entertain a plan to remember his name and return with a gift for him.

In the endless hospital scenes of my childhood, I played the stoic. They would tell me I could scream if I wanted, but it was easy not to. I can't recall ever making a peep. They were impressed and approving when I could be pricked any number of times and respond only with a little frown and a polite smile. I never protested, even though I looked even younger than I was. I was smarter than the other kids who didn't understand that if you objected, it would only take longer before it was over. You weren't getting out of it anyway. And if you annoyed them they wouldn't be as kind to you, or as gentle doing it.

I was an endless receptacle for pain. It would feel as if I was being torn apart, puking and crying, and soon after my parents would send me walking to school like any other kid. I was an infinite resource, endlessly flexible. No consequences, just a chain of exhausting school days, punctuated by trying to stall having to go to bed alone in my bedroom. My sister was kept out of it. My parents, a nurse and a doctor, would say that being sick only meant there was all the more reason to be good. I was different than other kids, so I needed to be more careful, smarter, and tougher. One part was them acting as if what they wished—that I would be healthy and happy—was simply true. Another part included toughening me up, which they thought I would need—and children will rise to almost any level that is demanded of them. Yet another was part making sure that my illness didn't "control our entire family", that I wouldn't be able to manipulate my way to advantages and extra attention, just because I was sick.

So, I was often left to cope with the trouble and pain all by myself. I tried to hide my illness and be as charming as possible about it when I couldn't. Being tough and brave was the way to get their approval and some comforting. I have a hard time forgiving the fact that the shame and loneliness that isolated me was convenient for them.

In the bright ER cubicle after midnight, it's dark outside the partition curtains. The bed is in the center of the room, with a sink and shelves covered in little boxes of equipment lining the walls. I'm in bed, still wearing my own pajama pants; the scuffed knee I often finger is there in front of me, out of reach. Neither lying down nor sitting up is okay, so I'm somewhere in between, sliding down into a more prostrate position. Kjetil occasionally gets up and grabs me under my arms to gently pull me further up on the bed. We've been waiting for hours for a doctor to come see me.

Kjetil appears to relish the thought of going to find someone to battle with, bringing a doctor back by force if he has to. I don't comment. We are both in doubt about whether I can be left alone. The nurses who come and go keep asking me for a urine sample and Kjetil wheels me back to the bathroom. It's a long way down the hall and involves an awkward and uncomfortable trip in and out and of an ER wheelchair designed to hold someone with an ass five times the size of mine. I have to use my ragged stomach muscles to remain on the jiggly seat, and Kjetil has trouble navigating it at the same time as the IV stand. When we finally get to the dimly lit bathroom I lean against the walls and go through all the necessary preparations but then I can't go this time either, just like last time. I take a minute to check out my sorry state in the mirror and see if I'm going to cry. No, just one sob, and then my dull eyes look back at me again.

Back in the cubicle, Kjetil keeps standing up, pacing, and sitting down, but still manages to appear calm. He keeps examining the equipment in the room. There is so much of it. Large machines attached to the walls. We can't divine the purpose of any of them. Every time our eyes meet he has his gentle smile ready for me, in case I want it.

I have at some point this last year finally begun to realize that it doesn't do me any good to be quiet and polite. This represents a paradigm shift, the whole world tilting thirty degrees and everyone just going about their day as if nothing happened. It doesn't do me any good to pretend I'm not angry when I am, despite what my parents told me I had to do to get what I need: be a good, appealing patient, because no one cares and no one wants to be bothered. Doctors and nurses can't stop treating me even if I were to be rude to them. In fact, being demanding might even get me more attention and better care. It's been so many years of holding myself back that I am in danger of turning into one of those terrifying people who can transmit their darkness, their anger and misery in every single way except out loud, in words. Because apparently, even though I am clamping down on it, anyone with eyes can tell I am furious. I am enraged, I'm raining fire, smashing bridges against skyscrapers and raising my throat to the sky to sound a yell that will have all the windows in the city crashing to the ground in lethal shards.

The body in the bed. They have sheathed it in a hospital shirt and given it a little plastic bag with a plastic ring around the opening to throw up in. I hold onto it even though it's been hours since I last vomited. I squeeze the firm plastic ring between my fingers. Silence isn't an effort anymore, it's a natural state. Some percentage of me is made of stone.

But now I'm moaning loudly, and every time the pain comes back I kick and kick the sheets. There is less than a minute of pause between the intense waves of pain, and always a steady, queasy buzz beneath them. Groaning is a tiny bit better than being quiet. It's somewhat comical to allow all kinds of noise to escape my mouth unchecked. I wonder if I am benefiting from not spending that energy on being still. Maybe it is actually an expenditure of energy to make sounds instead. Lifting the maze, allowing all the rats to run wild, scratching the floors frantically, crazily climbing on top of each other to spread chaos in every direction like an undulating siren, letting you know that there is a crisis! *What will keep the world from falling apart if I'm just an empty, moaning rag doll in a bed, not a giant made of stone with endless powers of control, towering over the city? Is there any energy in me at all if not the one that comes from being under pressure?* If any of this were to be looked at straight on instead of sideways and tilted, if I were to actually realize how much trouble I'm in, my life would fall apart. Even more than it already has. I laugh a tiny little laugh that goes unnoticed.

Kjetil sits down on a stool with wheels and holds my hand in between his. The openness of his face has always been a gift. His warm eyes, like he will accept whatever I give him, even treasure it. He is well-dressed, well-educated, and kind. How lucky I am to have someone like that, who offers himself up for use, to pour any excess misery onto—and even though that is only a little bit possible, I deeply appreciate this gesture. He looks at me intently, but reassuringly. I wish I could somehow meditate on how sunlit he is, the daylight he brings to this room. But I can't. I'm stuck inside myself. I gasp, kick, moan.

A new wave of pain comes and it's worse than before. Kjetil stands up, in alarm. The room is still, everything here is fixed and real. I am the one sliding, going, metamorphosing. I am completely trapped, here and now.

I watch my frail plans for the future circle the drain. There's been a nonstop radio broadcast in my head that keeps repeating that this is what it'll be like from now on, pure darkness. *Every little problem, every run of the mill stomach bug will turn huge and impossible and bring us here, where I can't breathe from fear. The rest of my life will be like this, there'll never be more than a week at a time without a major disaster. There is no place to go. I have no power over anything. I'm at the mercy of strangers who don't listen and can't see me. My life shrinks and shrinks, gets worse and worse, while more and more parts of my body will fail with increasingly humiliating results, results so awful I can't even imagine them yet.*

The logical end to all this is death, the ultimate felling of the body, bowels releasing, and tongue rolling out, the soft parts of the body hardening and the hard parts softening, everything opposite of how it should be, an extinguishing of this body—this one, these pale hands slightly yellow in the fluorescent light, these pink nails with the ragged cuticles. It's real and it's true: this body is all I am, the only place in the world I can be. From now on there is no way out, even for a second.

I moan.

"That's enough, I'm going to find someone," Kjetil says angrily. He runs into a heavyset, middle-aged nurse with a beehive hairdo, right outside the curtain.

"Someone has to come look at her! This is insane!"

She's unimpressed. "Everyone here needs a doctor. Someone will be with you soon."

After I cry for a little while, I stop and stare into the air, feeling the layers for an iota of improvement. Crying, kicking, waiting, groaning.

A surgeon comes and examines my swollen stomach. I don't have an appendix after the last surgery, so that's not it. He flips through the surgical notes, all six pages.

"How long after the surgery did you have a colostomy?" he asks.

"I've never had a colostomy."

"Really? Lucky."

This gives me pause. I never knew I was close to a colostomy situation.

He doesn't think I'm his domain because he thinks it's a virus. The internist takes her time. The nurse with the beehive hairdo gives me two paracetamols. They want to see if I get worse without the symptoms masked by drugs. It's like trying to put out a house fire with a moist towelette, but for some reason it seems to work a little. The pain lessens a bit and I regain a little of myself. These territories are right under the surface of daily life.

Everything is okay as long as I'm not in pain.

The internist comes and goes, and like everything else we wait for, she brings no real change, just the next stage of waiting. Still there is relief and comfort in having a place to go. The nurses after my biggest surgery had tricks that helped, like pulling the duvet down to my hips and then laying a baby blanket over my torso because it weighed less on my wounds. They persuaded me to shower on the third day. I took ages, slowly washing in the clean babyish scent of the super-mild hospital soap. When I came back, they'd made up the bed with fresh sheets and tucked me in gently after changing my bandages.

My pulse is too high, so the internist orders an EKG when she finishes with a thorough cross-examination. The beehive nurse wheels the apparatus in. Kjetil perks up a little at the sight of it; he's always interested in how machines work. The nurse opens the top of my shirt and prepares the skin on my chest, first with a wipe, and then drying it with gauze. There are so many wires. We watch her sorting them methodically.

"How can you keep them straight?" Kjetil asks. She is wearing blue eye shadow and has a slight Russian accent. Her face is round and seems friendly now. She smiles.

"It's tricky. Everyone has their own verse for remembering the order. Mine is like a description of the world…I start at the bottom. The red one is the center of the earth. It goes here…" She places the cool and moist electrode cushion on my chest. Her fingers are light on my skin. Kjetil is leaning over me a little, his eyes are fixed on her motions.

"The brown one is the earth…here," she places another one.

"The blue one is the ocean, here…The green one is the trees and plants…the yellow one, here, is the sun in the sky, where the white one is the clouds, and this last, purple one is the stars, the Milky Way."

I look up at Kjetil, who's smiling eagerly at her while she talks. And there it is, an impulse I have never understood before: *I want to protect him from all this.*

I come from a family of hard-asses, but I've never understood their desire to push any support or tenderness away. I may not know exactly how to deal with it, but I've always craved it. There has always been a poverty of all of that. When characters in books and movies heroically and romantically make gestures to protect others, and stoically send away help, I find it ridiculous and infuriating. No one in real need would ever do such a thing—only a bullshit character invented by a privileged, romanticizing ass would ever reject help and love in a situation of desperate need. Am I supposed to believe an injured soldier would say, "No, no, put me down! Leave me here to die alone in the jungle!"? What sort of patient would tell her lover to not come back and visit, to forget her? Wouldn't you want to get out of the damp Victorian hospital where all cures make you worse? Don't you want a life? Can't you see that their healthy bodies are solid, made from different stuff than yours—that what it costs them is much less than what it is worth to you? They could brighten your life much more than you could darken theirs. What sort of idiot are you?

So, I am learning something. Here it is: I want to protect him. I want to keep him out of this awful situation that my life has become. The responsibility is too big a burden. I don't want to need him like this. *I don't want this.*

I don't think my way to this conclusion. It arrives, and it will come with me upstairs. I'll look at it sometime later. I'll do what I have to do.

They wheel me upstairs and place me in the corridor because the ward is full. I fall asleep hearing the rain on the roof, using Kjetil's plaid shirt that smells like him to cover my eyes because the gentle nurses can't figure out how to turn off the hallway lights.

Lutz: A difficult jump that requires a long, gliding buildup. The skater is exerting force against the natural body movement; the jump is approached clockwise but is performed counterclockwise.

The door to my room opens a crack, I get a glimpse of the nurse, and then the bottle of hand cream I've asked for is kicked through the door. It lands near the bed. She has momentarily forgotten her professionalism and just solved the problem in the most obvious way—transferring an object into the isolation room without touching anything. When she catches my eye, she's embarrassed. She pokes her blonde head through the door, holding the facemask in place with her gloved hand.

"I got a little carried away there. Sorry...I'll see about getting you that TV."

I've already gotten out of bed and picked up the lotion. My hands are raw from all the hand washing I've been doing. Everything I touch feels unpleasant.

To enter my room, visitors must first put on blue disposable pants, which look like paper on the outside but are plastic on the inside. Over that goes a long yellow plastic coat with strings tied around the waist, blue elastic slippers over their shoes, face mask, hat, and lavender vinyl gloves. When my plastic-sheathed guests enter the room, I see sweat begin to bead on the exposed inches of skin on their foreheads. They very quickly wish they could leave. The outfits are only ever worn for a few minutes, and when they come off, a single one fills a whole trash bag, which needs to be sheathed in another bright yellow one before being removed according to the rules. Only Kjetil wears his for hours, sweating. Every evening he stays until his yawns become too frequent. He brings food, so I won't have to chance the hospital kitchen's allergy routines. He works, comes home, cooks, packs up the food, takes one bus and then another, and then walks around the hospital grounds to find to me.

The isolation room is large for one bed, comfortable and freshly decorated. I come to kind of love it. I'm still in pain, staggering between the bathroom and the bed. But there's also a dog-tired peace of sorts. I feel considerable relief at not having to share my precious toilet with anyone, and at how clean everything is.

Nothing is expected of me here. My endless to-do list and the sucking vortex of anxiety about my future remains outside the sluice door, along with everything else. Any talk about what will happen next has been paused completely. I tell Kjetil to remind me of my new realization that *it is better not to worry. It will be the exact same moment without the worry.*

Gastrointestinal specialists are kinder than surgeons. They've settled it being a virus, because they can't find any other explanation—a run of the mill stomach virus, the complications of overactive nerves and an extremely sore and irritable digestive system and the other pain because of the recent surgery.

I'm alone with my virus.

It gives me some pleasure that the color combination of the visitors' protection outfits actually matches the isolation room itself—lemon yellow walls, pale lavender floor, and the curtains that have both colors and add a perfectly harmonizing stripe of moss green to the mix. As Norwegian institutional aesthetics go, it's a miracle of loveliness. I slowly pace the room in an ongoing attempt to ease my abdominal cramps, steering my IV stand awkwardly. The bathroom floor is a delicate lilac color with actual specks of glitter—God knows how the person who designed the room got away with that.

I encounter my pallid puffy-eyed self again in the mirror. *I don't look too bad. Lost a little weight, brings out the cheekbones.* The crimson pout of my sore lips, a careless gaze, like a model in a fashion magazine, I think. The almost-bruised rings around my eyes enhance the effect, sort of. The blue hospital shirt, not so much. I turn and shuffle back to bed until I can manage a repeat. I sleep as much as I can and when I get a TV on the second day I watch hour after hour of reality shows about people learning new skills and getting makeovers. It's the only thing on that I can follow. I find it quite satisfying.

The view from my room is of an enormous chimney, taller than the hospital building I'm in. There's also a stretch of lawn that has been left to its own devices. Wildflowers and tall stalks of grass spread their seeds from gracile fingers. There's a gravel walking path no one ever seems to use. The pale blue sky never darkens completely, though it's August. There's a sloping mountain in the distance. It's quiet, but I can hear birds. There's no noise from within the ward either, because of the extra sluice door.

I look out the window and wait.

A week before my departure date to New York, they let me go. I have a bone scan my doctor has ordered as a precaution—a starting point to measure the potential long-term damage against, since I'll be on injections that undermine bone density for the foreseeable future. Despite the nasty side effects to my skeleton and elsewhere, the injections are the only real way to regulate the pain from the endometriosis. The technician tells me the results will take two weeks, but that very same day at 6 p.m., my young GP calls, right after I've come through the door at home. She informs me I have a pre-stage of osteoporosis. I lean against the fridge and grit my teeth. I'll need to come in and talk to her about it. I'll need to decrease my cortisone asthma medicine to reduce the damage.

I'll need a lung specialist in New York as soon as I arrive to find a reduced dose, I learn. I have to take high doses of vitamin D and calcium. I should be running and lifting weights several times a week to rebuild my bone density. My brain crackles. I'm dizzy from climbing the single flight of stairs to my apartment. I've been skipping the calcium tablets—precautionary until now—because they make me nauseous: now I have to take four a day for the rest of my life. I might need to take stronger medication, the osteoporosis drug my aunt takes that makes her feel like she has the flu for two days after each monthly dose.

Kjetil arrives home to reassure me that everything will be okay. I've been crying and my eyes are swollen. I keep pulling at my hair so it stands straight up and I've rolled up my shirt and fastened it under my bra because it still hurts to have fabric weighing on my stomach. I'm wearing my sister's old, unflattering pregnancy jeans, the soft, stretchy waist rolled down in bunches below my hip-bones. I catch a glimpse of myself in the mirror: I look crazy.

Kjetil loosens his tie and drops down on the couch, a dog-tired expression on his face. I have no reserves left to wonder what he's thinking. A sort of heat impinges on my thoughts and it becomes impossible to think; I can offer nothing but muttered curses and crying. How long will he stand for this? *I can't live without him*. But I know I wouldn't die. Even suicide is no solution. *Soon I'll be out of his life and I won't be responsible for that tired and unhappy face anymore, won't be wondering how long I can keep him. His life would be better without me, I can't have him, just like I can't have anything*. I have to take his help now because I can't survive without it, but if I get out of here, if I manage to leave, I'll let him go. The thought comes with a bitterness that almost chokes me, but for a second I feel the cool touch of relief, too, a touch of power.

Everything on my to-do list is checked off. I've boarded the plane, sat down, belt fastened, we are in the air. *It's better not to worry.* I can barely sit still, though I'm exhausted. I wouldn't be surprised if the plane burst into flames right now. On the other hand, this is it—a few hours to rest and enjoy before more work, lists, and fears.

On the other side of the Atlantic, a clean, furnished studio apartment awaits me. The best 40 percent of my clothes will be folded tidily in the drawers: new shampoos, fancy organic soaps and lotions that I'll enjoy choosing and paying for in dollars will be lined up neatly in the bathroom. Everything in the apartment will be small, well-thought-out, and mine. There will be a lock and chain on the door and no one can come in unless I invite them.

New York's rosy yellow hue will seem golden compared to the cooler colors of home. The air will be soft, thick and warm. The whiff of strangers' sweat and of surprising perfumes will trail after them in the constantly moving crowds on the subway steps. Bright earrings and perfect manicures will catch my eye. There will be the scent of sturdy leaves and flowers from strange trees, and of something fresh and sweet in the air as I make my way across the uneven stone paths of campus. There will be books to read and classes to attend a manageable six-minute walk from my apartment. Everyone will be friendly and polite, and no one will know who I am.

For now, there is only the blue sky outside the plane.
Nothing but an enormous, perfect absence.
I fall asleep.

PART 5

ONE MORE TIME WITH FEELING

2009

Doctors barely hear what you say. They watch your demeanor and listen for the tone of your voice. If you're too hysterical, they write you off. If you're too calm, they do the same. You must:

- appear sympathetic
- make them realize you're a human being, just like them
- be self-deprecating enough to make it clear that you don't take yourself too seriously
- preferably make them laugh
- make sure they see that your symptoms are real
- state your problems concisely so they don't feel like you're wasting their time
- but squeeze all relevant information in at once
- never wait for them to ask the questions that lead to the pertinent stuff, or it'll never come up
- never assume they understood you
- never cry
- or, maybe you should cry?

Is it like this for men, too? Despite my intense efforts to master this system, to present myself exactly the right way to get what I need and want, I can't seem to do it right.

The first time I mention the increased abdominal pain to my new GP—a young woman with short hair—we've been living in Oslo for a month, ever since Kjetil started his first real job here. I'm officially looking for work.

"If this was anything that needed attention you would be kicking me in the face right about now for being so rough," she says, smiling, and applying pressure to my stomach while I'm on my back. I like her. I'm just frowning a little, my jaw tight, hazily worried. Looking up at her, I wonder what level of discomfort warrants a reaction—the pain that is there the whole time, all over, or only the peaks. *How big should the peaks be?* I already told her I have pain. *What is the right response—do I try to make it sound like an authentic outcry* (Ow!), *or just a calm word of notification* (Yes. There.)*?* There's a delay to my reactions. Something slides silently to seal the exits, to keep whatever it is inside. Before I can identify a difference in sensation, her hands move on to a different spot and it seems easier to not say anything. It's over so quickly I barely make a sound.

I'm applying to American graduate schools. One of my friends assures me that I actually have a chance of getting in. I don't believe it, but there's nothing better for me to spend my time on, between medical appointments and scanning listings for jobs I'll never get. I've been ready for a change for a while, but it turns out that staying inside our small apartment writing all day long is less fun than I pictured when I was still working at the tourist information center in Bergen. I don't feel well, either. I've recovered from the move, but I still feel exhausted all the time, despite not really doing anything. Kjetil often cooks dinner and does the grocery shopping, even though he works long hours, because I can't find energy to do it—though I'm ashamed. All my regular problems like painful muscles and stomachaches are in a rough patch that never seems to pass. My skin looks terrible.

All my life, there have been bad, sometimes horrible rough patches that eventually end. I wait for it to pass on its own. I try to exercise as much as I can.

The thought of going to school in the US and changing my whole career, taking a stand for myself as an artist, is unbelievably exciting. It feels dangerous, too, as if I couldn't possibly effect this much change in my life. The last few years have been full of nice memories—living a normal life alongside Kjetil, who makes everyday life fun. Work, friends, parties. Writing on days off. When I look back, though, I see I haven't done that much besides get older. I enjoy having to work hard to finish the applications.

Kjetil is a happy person, generally untroubled by the world. I'm finally old enough to appreciate that rare quality for what it is and the benefits of it for me, rather than resenting his privileged life. He's kind, funny, and willing to see things from others' perspectives, and take time to think things through. I spent quite a lot of time convincing him that my world view is accurate before I realized I could borrow some of his, too. When I look at the world through his eyes, it seems believable that more things might actually be alright than not. The future *can* hold good things. I *can* enjoy life. There's sad and horrible stuff in the world, but you don't have to go looking for it—or at least, I don't. I'm allowed to have fun. I can have a life. I can be normal and healthy. I can write.

During summer and fall, though, pain slowly winds itself around my torso while I attempt to settle into life in Oslo. I grow aware of it gradually. Occasional bad days make an appearance and then become more frequent. For a long time, I hope the pain will simply go away, I try to shake it off like a cramp, but it clamps onto my entire left side, from my ribs to the top of my thigh, my spine to my navel. Then it spreads until it ropes around my right side. It's a familiar sensation long before it becomes predominant enough for me to have to notice it. The realization that something is not right has to strike me several times before I take any action. It's like waking up slowly to earsplitting noise. You can stay half-asleep for a long time, despite the walls ringing with it. Even though it barely affected you at all for a long time, once you hear it there's no way to un-hear it even for a second. You panic to make it stop.

I mail my last grad school application on an incredibly cold day in January. I can't close my jacket over my stomach because of the pain, so I wear an extra warm hat to compensate, but it doesn't work. My first surgery to remove two ovarian cysts that are presumably causing the pain is just days away. I'm in constant pain, but they're fixing me up. I'll be in great shape soon. Kjetil and a friend wait outside on the street, in the low sun, stamping on the creaky snow, cheeks bright red from the cold. The girl at the post office refuses to stamp the envelope to show that the application letter was mailed on time.

My attitude is that I can handle it. I've done hospitals and doctors before. There's still a subcutaneous layer of strength left. Kjetil doesn't come with me to the hospital. His work hours are still murderous. He takes his cues from me and there is no one else paying attention or giving advice. The first surgery is outpatient, a friend comes with me and leaves when I go in.

The operation reveals "deeply infiltrating endometriosis," which has worsened, unimpeded, for years. My entire pelvis and lower abdomen are inflamed, dense with scar tissue and adhesions from old bleeding, fusing my organs and twisting them. When I wake from surgery, there are two leaflets for me on my bedside table. One about endometriosis, the disease I didn't know I have: its symptoms, effects and related fertility problems. The other leaflet is about chronic pain. Looking at them, it's clear to me that I'm taking the pain home again.

The day after surgery is a Saturday. I'm glad, because Kjetil would have a hard time taking time off work, and I think I might need a little babysitting. We wake up together in bed and I feel good, much better than I expected, much better than I've felt lately. The bad news they gave me about my infiltrating endometriosis is still distant. There's hardly any pain. I'm elated. I'm done!

We cuddle and linger in bed before getting up to have breakfast. He uses the bathroom first and takes his time in there. When he gets out, I teeter towards the bathroom on unsteady feet. He asks if I want oatmeal. I'm already way too hungry. I sit down gingerly on the toilet, carefully clutching my swollen, bandaged stomach. I should've taken the pain pills they gave me before getting out of bed, because it's starting to hurt. A lot. I wondered how surgical wounds would feel and whether I would feel the cuts, but it just hurts, like something dark purple, darker in color further down on my stomach. There's a painful, twisting sensation in my shoulders and chest, like trapped wind. Now that I've noticed it, I can't stand it. My mother warned me,

"Your shoulders might hurt because of the gas they use during surgery," but this feels bizarre.

When I exit the bathroom, I smell an awful motor oil-like stench. The kitchen is only lit by the stove light. It's practically dark outside even though it's 10 a.m. Freezing Oslo January grimness. I'm wearing wool socks and wool longs under my pajamas and I'm still cold. An oily chemical is running all over the kitchen cabinet. The smell is noxious and so overwhelming I almost retch. Kjetil is standing on a chair in his boxer shorts, trying to wipe it from the kitchen cabinets with paper towels, managing to spread the viscous, gray fluid over the white surface.

"What's that horrible smell? Why is it so dark in here? Why haven't you made breakfast?"

My voice is loud and screechy.

"The kitchen light is dead. I was getting the light bulb from the top of the cupboard, and I knocked over the bottle of bike chain lube. I'm taking care of it, okay?" He is becoming atypically irritable in the face of my outburst.

"It smells horrible! I can't stand it! And I need to eat!" I start crying, angry, panicky tears running down my face. After that there's just an awful blur of my out of control voice and his cranky face, looking at me like I'm an unappealing stranger.

"Calm down. I'm taking care of it. I'll make breakfast in a minute, okay?"

Clearly, this is my cue to back off, but I can't.

"You took too long in the bathroom! I have to take my painkillers. Where are they?"

"I don't know, aren't they in your bag?"

"I don't know! I was on drugs! I can't eat with this smell! I'll throw up and rip my stitches!"

"Well, make up your mind, do you want me to make breakfast or clean this up?" He's getting loud, too.

"It's too cold to even open the windows! How am I going to spend the whole day in an apartment that stinks like this? Why aren't you helping me? Why are you being horrible instead of nice?" I sit down at the kitchen table and sob into my hands. He gets down from the chair and loudly puts the oatmeal on, banging the pot against the stove. He brings me a glass of water and my bag with the hospital pill envelope in it and tells me to swallow my pills. Then he holds me for a minute while I weep, without saying anything. He works on the spill for a long time with dishwashing detergent and paper towels, but the smell lingers in the apartment for days.

A few weeks go by before I go back to the hospital for an MRI. I haven't asked for any of the sedatives available for claustrophobic patients, not only because I don't think I am, but also because I'm attached to an image of myself as the perfect patient, someone who's been around the block.

This time, even my feet are inside the tiny space of the MRI machine, and the noise is shockingly loud and bizarrely rhythmic. It vibrates through my body and immediately activates an animal need in me to be out of there *now*. Over the din, the loud, scratchy, cheerful radio voices in my headphones turn into alien shrieking. All I can do is chant *Oh God, oh God, oh God* silently in my head, over and over. Through the headphones, the radiology nurse instructs me to "try not to breathe so much". He keeps stopping and starting over because, he says, my intestines are moving too much, despite the fact that I've been fasting since the night before. When he finally wheels me out of the MRI machine after an hour and a half, I can't keep it together a second longer. I curl into a ball, still on the stretcher, and gasp out one bleak, undignified sob after another. The nurse waits impatiently for me to finish so he can bring in the next patient, not saying a word.

"I think there's ice on that outdoor rink at Spikersuppa these days. It's free. Why don't you meet me there after work tomorrow and I can admire you while you skate?"

We're packing some stuff to put in our attic storage space, and Kjetil has caught me caressing the smooth, heavy leather of my skates.

"I've never seen you on the ice," he says, smiling. "I bet you'd look good."

He's being kind. I try to picture myself on the ice, but all I can think of are things that are lost forever. My bloated, clumsy, exhausted current body hovers over the image of my self-possessed, sleek inner teenage figure skater. Even the thought is humiliating. I'd rather have the unsullied memory of my body doing a beautiful thing, taking the tall, athletic boy I was in love with at the time to the quiet rink on a fall day off from school when I was sixteen, wearing the perfect outfit (tight jeans and a short, moss-green fitted sweater that brought out my eyes) as I jumped, pirouetted, and outraced him effortlessly. Seeing the admiration grow on his face as he chased after me, that look that meant he was dying to get his hands on me, our laughter echoing in the cool air of the nearly empty rink.

I smile faintly at Kjetil.

"Maybe next year."

Jump series: several jumps in succession, but with steps, turns, hops or changes of feet between the landing of one jump and takeoff of the next.

The MRI reveals that the disease is everywhere, including my intestines. There's a CT scan, countless doctors, more sonograms and consultations, and then they plan a second, complex procedure with multiple surgeons of different specialties to remove several parts of the intestines that are, in the surgeon's own words, "ruined". The surgery is also to extract as much of the endometrial tissue over my abdomen and pelvis as possible, to free the organs that are stuck to each other, while attempting to minimize the harm done to all my affected organs . I have to wait another three months for a surgery date when all the surgeons are available.

Gynecological surgeons are not typically known for their bedside manner. "Endometriosis is a bitch," one surgeon tells me with a sigh. "We know what happens but we don't know the causes; we can't stop it. Too much surgery makes it worse, the medications regulate it only partially and have bad side effects, but if we don't treat it, you'll get worse with every month."

My surgeon is one of Norway's prime specialists in the field of hopelessly under-researched female misery. It's probably a thankless career and it doesn't seem to sit very well with him.

His ego is always in the room and he does not enjoy having his authority questioned. He is always rushed, doesn't make much eye contact, and always cuts me off when I talk. In fact, he literally can't seem to hear me very well, and that annoys him. I write lists of questions and try to explain the complex situation in as few words as possible. I try to speak loudly and very clearly, but there is always a moment when he looks at me with irritated disbelief.

His voice curt, he says things like: "Well, you're just going to have to live with a certain level of pain."

He may not mean it unkindly, but it certainly comes across that way. Directly behind him in my line of vision, the accompanying nurse leans out of her chair and strains to make eye contact with me and hum empathetically. At the end of several appointments, the nurse chases after me in the hallway, asking if I'm all right while I try to make it to the bathroom to cry in peace.

"Oh dear, I know he can be a bit harsh," she says. "But he's a great surgeon."

I need this doctor on my side. If I spend my precious twenty minutes with him trying to change his behavior, it'll only hurt me. If I file a complaint, he'll know it was me.

I bring Kjetil along to an appointment and the doctor is having a good day for once. He seems pleasant and relaxed, asking what Kjetil does and even making time for some banter. After he's examined me, he keeps talking to Kjetil about me while I'm behind the partition getting dressed. I can't quite hear what they're saying, but he's talking about my prognosis.

When I come to sit down, I try to think his talking with Kjetil about me is only a misunderstanding. It's only because the appointment time is so short that the doctor has to make use of the moments when I'm getting dressed too. Or maybe he just got carried away. It must be a coincidence that he's so much nicer when Kjetil is here.

But then he does the same thing on my next visit, and the one after that.

After Kjetil starts carving out time in his schedule to come with me consistently, the entire dynamic shifts and I stop thinking of the doctor as someone akin to an enemy and start believing he is trying to help me as best he knows how.

One time, when Kjetil can't come with me, I dread the appointment even more than usual.

"You could wear a fake mustache and pretend you're him," Ingrid suggests. "He'll probably be thrilled to have Kjetil show up without you."

A few weeks before the second operation, I finally make it out of the house by myself. It's my friend Marius's twenty-ninth birthday. He moved to Oslo three years ago and knows a lot of very energetic people. I recently turned twenty-eight, but Kjetil and I haven't celebrated it yet. We still don't know that many people in Oslo.

Marius is already drunk when I arrive, and happy as a clam. He plants a loud, wet kiss on my cheek, puts a plastic cup in my hand and dances away down the hall. The kitchen is full of people, plastic bags, wine bottles, and beer. I hold the drink I probably shouldn't be drinking and try to smile and look friendly. There are only strangers around me, and one of them bumps me hard enough for me to almost lose my balance. He doesn't apologize. The music is loud and I'm already close to tears. I think I might just go home right away, if it weren't for the fact that Kjetil seemed so glad I was well enough to go out without him. He followed me to the door of our apartment to kiss me when I left, wearing an old hoodie and holding a bottle of some exotic beer in his hand, happy to have an evening home alone, for once. I think he misses being a student. We left most of our friends in Bergen when we moved.

I move so my back is to the wall, next to a windowsill with plants on it. Yesterday was a rough day and my eyes are still swollen and achy, having spent hours crying like I was getting paid for it. Earlier today, I had a nap and a very vivid dream in which I visited Veronica Mars and watched her dust a huge collection of old radios in a sunny room with a high ceiling. I wanted to stay there.

I tried on all my clothes before I left, but nothing I can wear these days is flattering. I am wearing a loose shirt I'm hoping makes me look stylish, if not pretty. My stomach is distended; it doesn't work with any outfit. I recently cut my hair, but it doesn't look the way I want it to, because my face doesn't look the way I want it to. It's swollen, and my back is hunched. I feel only barely within the region of *woman*. This is some other entity, a sexless uncharted territory between "old person" and "child". I've seen people like that on the street, overcome by the body so it seems like their eyes are looking out at you from somewhere deep inside. I can't show my skin to anyone. It's painful, flecked, red. One light layer of soft wool is too heavy, hurts and stings the body beneath.

I have no idea how to talk to people anymore. None of my friends have experienced anything similar enough to know what to say to me. I read their silences and stock phrases as signs that they can't wait for me to stop talking about my health.

Finally, someone shouts, “Laura! Is that you?!”

It’s a girl I went to school with years ago. She is heavily made-up and wearing a black dress with sequins and heels. Her eyes are glittery with eye shadow. She hugs me briefly.

“What do you do these days?” she yells in my ear after exclaiming at how great it is to see me. I evade the question and ask about her. She tells me that she and her husband have a house and two little boys. When she keeps asking about my life, the part of me that always wants to please people ends up embarrassedly telling her the abbreviated story of my illness. I cringe, I want to stop talking about it, but once I’ve started there is no way out.

“Oh no, you poor thing!” she cries. “If that happened to me, I would just have them yank everything out. I have two boys, you know! More than enough!” She laughs a little, her eyes look over my shoulder for someone else to talk to.

The call comes two weeks before my second surgery, informing me that I have a spot in the graduate degree writing program in New York City. We drink a little champagne to celebrate. Kjetil starts to look for work in New York so he can come with me. My head might explode from excitement, but I’m also desperate and scared stiff at how much I already need this. *I need a new world, where things aren’t ruined.*

When we were little, everything new, glamorous, and funny came from America. They rationed out the TV shows and films on the state channel like it was candy, as if too much of it would get in the way of proper nutrition. I can’t even picture it. It will be better, shinier than anything I can imagine. I need to be someone else, someone who can do something good and worthy.

I keep mobilizing all my energy to do just one more task within the last deadline, to make sure it won't be that one piece of paperwork that ruins my dream to move to New York. It takes all I have to maintain that effort through panic, pain, and a haze of painkillers that don't work. In the pre-surgical meeting, the surgeon mentions again that if I want children of my own, I'd better start planning now. I just look at him and he moves on quickly. As if I could ever do a single thing to risk this body again. As if I'm not already barely holding on. As if I've been doing womanhood wrong by being a person instead of a mother. As if I should choose pain, discomfort, hospitals, choose to be trapped in even more ways, choose my vulnerability personified outside of this body. As if I would choose this fucking body over my art. *As if I intend to stay.*

Leaving is a terrifying thought, too, but as I count down the days to my second surgery, I know it's crucial. I know without ever forming the words to myself or anyone else that I can't stand my life the way it is much longer. I know that if I don't have a way out I would rather die.

I'll go away and find a way to somehow force my life to be different. Everything else is irrelevant. *I can't stay.*

We're early and can't find a way to get inside the ward, so we end up spending twenty-five minutes on one of two hard blue institutional couches in the hallway by the elevators, looking out over Oslo through the vast windows. It's a beautiful, clear day. Two other women arrive a little while after us and take the other couch. The hospital smell is still new. I'm petrified. My teeth chatter in my mouth, stomach clenched; it's my third day on a liquid diet. I hold Kjetil's hand, but it doesn't seem to help. Panicked, barely formed thoughts skitter across my mind like cockroaches. I try to tell myself to think only small thoughts for now. *Just wait.*

I feel alienated from the two women on the other couch, who look like two versions of the same person. Roughly twenty-five years between them, their faces have been altered in a uniform way—maybe it's the bloated lips. They both have big breasts and platinum blonde hair piled high on top of their heads. The younger one is wearing a lot of makeup. I spent last night meticulously following the many pages of instructions the hospital sent, taking breaks to rest in between every step, trying to get it all done before my blood sugar fell again, when the orange juice—my last meal—ran out. Washing my entire body very thoroughly, not shaving anything—"*we will help you shave if that is necessary,*" the instructions said—not putting on any creams or hair products. It feels inappropriate to try to look pretty at a time and place like this.

Nobody speaks. At 7:01, a nurse opens the door, calls my name, and leads Kjetil and me into a room with two beds. The surgeon is there, sitting on the edge of the hospital bed, legs sprawled in an extremely relaxed manner. Twenty minutes later, I'm naked inside the green robes, and all of a sudden, it's time to say goodbye to Kjetil in the hallway. I'm crying, but I try to choke back the tears because I think maybe it's dangerous during the anesthetic process to have a stuffy nose. He hugs me tightly and smiles, which feels wrong. I realize he is just trying to reassure me, but I can't believe he can smile at a time like this.

He is the person closest to me in the world, but right now there's a chasm between us. I am completely alone.

Before long, I'm padding on sock feet four floors down a spiral staircase, following two nurses who chat to each other. I try to think it's lucky that I won't have to wait any longer, but I know it's because I'm shit out of luck. They do the most difficult surgeries first.

I have been awake on and off for a few hours and at some point, it became nighttime. The room is dark and Kjetil is gone. He encouraged me to eat a few crackers, even though I couldn't have been less interested in eating. I think I talked to my mother briefly on the phone. The older woman from the hallway this morning groans in the bed across from mine.

For some reason, I keep finding myself sitting up in the hospital bed like I'm about to go somewhere and address someone about something urgent. One minute I am fitfully asleep, dreaming endlessly that my bed is covered in heavy junk I have to organize or hide from nurses who wait impatiently for me to finish so they can get on with things.

"Quite a mess you got there," one of them keeps saying in the dream. I have to try to sort out the chaos, even though I'm so tired and keep losing track of what I'm doing.

Another minute, I'm upright and talking, sort of awake, aware that I have been for a while. It's hard to calm down even though I am moving through molasses.

"Are you in pain?" I ask the groaning woman from this morning. I'm surprised at how steady my voice is, as if I'm a normal person. She says she doesn't want to bother the nurses and keeps getting out of bed to amble aimlessly around the furniture in the dark room, hunched over and still groaning. Her blonde hair gleams in the dimness. She is wearing a white T-shirt and the hospital underpants that look like the sheer tops of white pantyhose and don't actually constitute clothing.

To sit up in the bed, I have to lean back on my hands. I'm distantly aware that it should hurt more because there is a two-inch plastic needle in one of my wrists, but I can't feel a thing. It will be months before I can move with this kind of ease again; I still have no idea what state I'm in below the thick layer of drugs.

I tell the woman that's why the nurses are here. She still doesn't want to call them. Our communication is like my dreams, looping, no beginning or end. Still, we express a lot of friendly intent. She speaks to me in a soft voice, calls me tender names that are clearly translated from a different language. I finally press the call button and point to her when the nurse arrives. She gets a painkiller.

The night is endless. It doesn't take long before she's moaning again. This morning, while I was in the bathroom, I overheard her talking a nurse into letting her keep her own T-shirt instead of the hospital shirt, because it was more flattering. *Couldn't it at least be a normal person*, I thought. Now the thought of passing this night alone in a dark room is unthinkable. I don't mind her constant noises, how unaccustomed she is to how things work here. We are in this together, even though her surgery was much lighter than mine.

She tells me she's been sick for a while. She grew up in Spain. She tells me she left Spain to be a singer. She sings a little for me in Spanish. Her voice is deep and beautiful. The younger woman she was with yesterday is her daughter. She informs me that the daughter has a fluffy little dog called Bombón, which means chocolate, but also cutie, and that he is super, super cute. An issue of a men's magazine came out today with the daughter on the cover. She showed her mother a picture of it on her cell phone earlier. I have a vague memory of a smiling, blonde presence. At the time, I was barely conscious. I kept pulling my bangs straight up again and again and there was glue of some kind on my forehead. I kept chewing my lips. My roommate's voice brims with love and pride for her daughter.

She says Kjetil seems to love me very much. She is surprised that I am older than her daughter.

"So young to have this much trouble! Poor baby."

Her voice is warm. It's the most comforting thing I've heard in months.

There are long silences in between every exchange and we can only see each other when she is out of bed and moving around. I have a catheter and won't leave my bed for a couple of days yet. We go through another round of me calling the nurse for her, and I get another dose of anti-nausea medication, a cold little shower up my wrist. I can't believe how terrible I feel because I appear so at ease, even to myself. I should rest, I know, but falling asleep feels both dangerous and impossible. I keep checking my phone; the process of unlocking it so it will show me the time takes ages. 1:32 a.m. We are less than halfway through the night. Finally, the night nurse gives me a Valium. I sleep for almost three hours in one go. When I wake up, it's light outside and someone has moved the partition so I can see that my roommate is putting on mascara.

"I hated that they said not to wear makeup," she says. Her doctor comes in and she gets him to lean in, giggling. He's the surgeon from my first surgery, but he doesn't seem to remember me. The nurses are exasperated with her and think she is a disturbance to me. After the doctor's visit, they move me to a different room. As I'm wheeled away, she yells "Good luck! Adiós, guapa!"

Coming through the door of the hospital room, there Kjetil is finally, and my face slowly arrives in his neck, against his soft shirt collar under his suit. I smell the cologne we picked together and the scent of his skin. There is a little trace of fresh air on his clothes. His cheek is cold against mine. Our apartment is out there, along with the streets and trees and people moving around on their own, in control and in their own clothes, not even thinking for a second that it could be different. You can't see it while you're in it, only from further down the line, when life has become more broken. There is always more room further down, always more to lose that you didn't realize you had.

May is a warmer, sunnier month. The city is still mostly bare after the winter. My parents don't seem very concerned when they visit—first my mother, then my father. I may be reading them wrong. My mother's stay is a blur. They may be trying to help by not acknowledging that my situation isn't too fabulous. It's a seamless continuation of how they did it when I was little, when we all had our parts worked out. Maybe they're still saving some reserves for when things get even worse. Still, I want them to be worried, even shocked. I want half a sentence that expresses it.

I put on my big, puffy down jacket that doesn't squeeze my abdomen and my father and I inch down the stairs to take the world's slowest stroll around our backyard, me hanging on to his arm. We're lucky to have a big green backyard that we share with several unseen neighbors who lovingly tend to it. We see a cat and try unsuccessfully to lure it over. My father is quiet. I'm quiet.

Back inside, sunshine streams through the windows, and I sit up on the couch, which has been turned into a bed for me because I take several naps a day and I can't sit for long. My father does the dishes. It is day two out of the hospital, day six after the surgery. I'm on heavy-duty painkillers that keep a faint, sheepish smile on my face. My aunt Elsa sent me a multicolored ranunculus bouquet, which is displayed on the table. I can smell the flowers from here; the anesthesia has enhanced my sense of smell. It's like having acquired a superpower, which is somehow fitting. Last night I tried to eat a tiny piece of dark chocolate, but it was so strong and bitter that I spat it out in my hand, making a face like a baby. Kjetil and my father laughed at me. My father made a meal of potatoes, carrots and cod with salt and pepper, and I ate a miniscule portion. The delicate tastes had a complex range and were wonderfully delicious.

In the hospital, my sister sent a bouquet of three peonies that slowly opened over the course of three days and released a clean, glorious scent I could almost see (pale pink, laced with gold). I wasn't even aware that peonies had a scent, even though they're my favorite. The living room is quiet, except for the soft sound of water running in the kitchen sink. I'm trying to remember what I usually think of, and find that the baseline—which for months has been dread for the upcoming surgery—no longer applies. *It's over for now.* I have survived. It's like having survived a plane crash—a piece of spectacular bad luck and pain that rips you from everything that holds you, but returns you to where you were before you took off, to look around at what was. Well, it's like surviving with a partially broken body.

I think: *From now on I'm allowed to do whatever I want.*

PART 6

KEEP ON LIVING

2006

I'm on sick leave, even though it's only a summer job. I have regular appointments with a psychomotor physical therapist each Tuesday. My doctor has been filing paperwork for a year's extended sick leave for me to receive more treatment and see how I fare. Although it feels more physical than mental, my doctor informs me they'll only approve it if she argues that I have depression and psychosomatic stomachaches, since I'm only twenty-five. I'm still going to work, only fewer and shorter days. No one knows but my parents.

The trip to the physical therapist takes all the energy I have for a whole day. I take the bus to the center of town and then walk the last twenty minutes. There are no bus lines that go all the way there, and no bathrooms available along the second half of the walk, only deserted looking maritime businesses. My stomach often chooses to have a tantrum while I cover those insufferable kilometers. I hurry as much as humanly possible but walk in a very steady rhythm to lullaby my stomach. I must look ridiculous.

By the time I arrive, I'm sweaty and exhausted, rushing through the door, trying to organize my wet umbrella and my bag, yanking my headphones out of my ears to politely greet the receptionist. On lucky days, I'm only three minutes late, even though I try to leave some time to use the bathroom before I get called in. That means unlocking and relocking two doors down the hall, and it's freezing in there—so sometimes, I try to just sit very still to see if the cramps will calm down and I won't have to use the bathroom.

I prefer not to acknowledge what it was—*a fucking crisis*—when I come back from the bathroom and see Kari's open door waiting for me, but then it'll just seem like I was late again. And of course, I was. Ever since I started school, my mother has been repeating that I have to schedule in pockets of time to have a stomachache, so I won't always be late. During a rough patch in my childhood, she used to wake me up an hour early so I could have breakfast and my insides would have some time to calm down before walking to school. I've been relatively healthy the last six or seven years.

Kari's office is a simple room, painted blue, with a desk, chair, and massage table inside. I sit down on the chair. Kari is an athletic woman in her fifties with a broad smile and short, graying hair. She sits by her desk on an orthopedic balancing stool, her feet planted far apart on the floor. There are several photos of her on the wall above her desk, smiling against blue skies on mountaintops with other superhumans.

After a brief silence, during which I look at the encouraging posters on the walls, she asks me a brisk question about my week and I start to speak. The walk out here has shaken loose all the stuff I needed to talk about and none of it seems urgent or interesting anymore. I have to figure out how to talk as if it's never been done before, and she has to demonstrate again that she truly is interested by asking many follow-up questions.

Kari gives good, no-nonsense advice, but it's during the physical part of the treatment that the intense stuff happens. I might manage to be funny, insightful, and wise when we talk, only to become a mute moron when she asks me to do something specific with my body and tell her how it feels. Even with all the yoga I've been doing.

"As a psychomotor physical therapist, I don't chase particular pains around, because they move. I focus on the entire body to change your approach and give awareness, support, or stimulation."

I often have terrible pain in my arms and shoulders from work, sex, and too much time at the computer. I'm desperate to get rid of it, which is why I'm here, week after week. Sometimes I feel like she's sentencing me to another week in this pain. She only moves the painful muscle a bit, tests it, and then leaves it. I want her to trap it, grind it down, pierce it, force it to change. I don't care about approaching it carefully or with respect or *feeling it*. I'd rather bleed than keep feeling this particular frozen pain. Sometimes, I get nauseous when she works on my arms.

There's something about being in my underwear in a room with a medical professional that makes me shut down. I become dead meat. I hand myself over and vacate the premises. Afterwards, I don't even remember what happened. I might be able to dredge up some facts if pressed, but it's all in a part of my mind where someone has draped sheets over the furniture and turned off the light. I can get through almost anything. But I would like, at some point, to stop waiting out long stretches of my life. This is what Kari works on: getting me to own my body and remain inside it, getting me to realize that I can act according to what my body tells me. *I can take up some space.*

Under her guidance, I roll my spine gently up and down, bending and stretching my legs and arms. I work on breathing into my back and deep into my stomach, letting the air flow instead of holding my breath and tensing up my stomach, squeezing the air in and out with effort.

At the end of each session, I lie on my back underneath a blanket. It should be simple: she massages each leg gently, thigh first, then bends my knee and puts my foot on the table before moving on to my calf. She finds a spot between my calf muscles that's always sore or ticklish. Theoretically, the patient should, when experiencing the discomfort, kick the leg out, thus letting the physical therapist know that it's unpleasant, to stop. Kari immediately removes her hands and holds them up when I do, so it's a tiny and scheduled rebellion, the setting of a very small boundary. I have the worst trouble with this exercise and for the longest time could only do it by pretending: she would get to the point where I knew she expected me to kick and I would sort of fake a kick. Then she would tell me to do it properly and I would. I needed the explicit order each time.

I seem to take a long detour before I act on how I feel. It's not that I don't feel the pain. I do immediately. I just freeze up. Everything in me tells me to just wait a little and see if it passes so I won't have to do anything, won't have to inconvenience anyone, won't have to start over with the painful stuff. You'd think that once I identified this and consciously decided that protecting myself from discomfort outranks changing someone else's plan, I would be able to change my behavior, but no. It didn't fall away solved, like a knot when you tug the right string. The best I can do is dig trenches and establish habits with endless repetition and deliberate effort.

After that, she lifts each limb and tucks it inside the blanket and then I can finally let go of it and relax. She finishes the massage by lifting my head and stretching and massaging my neck very gently. She quietly smoothens my forehead with her fingers, places the palms of her hands on my scalp softly for a few seconds, then turns off the lights and leaves me to rest for a few minutes.

Those minutes after she leaves me are the most peaceful ones of my entire week. I try to let myself melt completely. I picture myself inside a healing and cleansing light, like my yoga teacher says to do during the guided meditation at the end of a class. I feel things slowly getting a little better. Each time, I cleanse my body a little more. It's like throwing out a toxic old fridge or an abandoned, moldy couch—I'm letting sunlight in.

After each session, no matter the weather, I go out to the tip of Nordnes Park, sit on a bench, and write in my notebook, looking at the sea through the metal railing. Even if I'm completely drained, I feel calm and present, a good kind of heavy. I rest in that sore feeling of having cried, of having uncovered something and seen what it is, and now being able to put it away a little. I breathe the fresh sea air deep into my lungs and think hopeful thoughts. Change doesn't just feel possible, it's actually happening.

I've just come gasping and depleted out of a bad year, in which my parents divorced and took turns going crazy. It gave me vertigo to see my strict, disciplined parents in despair, both of them crying over the phone and openly doubting every single choice they'd ever made. My mother has been on sick leave for months and talks constantly about how poor she is when living only off her own income. My sister Ingrid, who's married, had a whole different approach to our parents in crisis: "I'll spend time with them, but they should sort out their own crap." I didn't think I owed my parents much in the line of listening to their feelings either, since they raised us without doing much of that for us, but it was hard to avoid. It made me feel ill to see them suffer—although, now it's easier to talk to them, in a way; no one can pretend to be in control of anything, anymore. I've lost all patience for sad, droopy people to a point where they make my skin itch. I want to eat up all the sweetness I can find while it's in front of me. All those years, my parents really didn't know any better than I did.

Things have been picking up since the warm summer weather arrived at the beginning of June. I discovered the perfect haircut (short and tousled). I started yoga and have been slowly reclaiming my body through it three times a week, even before the physical therapy. Sleeping with Siri hasn't hurt either. I'm proud of my perfectly toned stomach and I've become one of those people who claim yoga can solve any problem. It even seems to help a little with the terrible menstrual pain that bends me in half every month. On those days I go pale and dizzy from the pain, even with painkillers. When I started yoga, I hadn't done anything with my body in years; it didn't even feel like it belonged to me. It was just something I'd been saddled with; uncooperative, painful, stiff, and embarrassingly weak. In the beginning, taking it through Ashtanga yoga was like trying to wrestle clothes onto a rigid mannequin in a tiny store window with people looking on.

I'm still more exhausted than other people ever seem to get. I try to accept what I feel, even if it's not jolly all the time. I take ages in the supermarket choosing the exact food I want to eat. Once I become aware of it, I'm amazed to realize how often I've denied myself little pleasures, even when the consequences were minimal. I listen intensely to music. I write poems and long journal entries. I'm making connections, digging, finding enormously heavy bullets to take back to Kari the next week. For little pockets of time inside her office, saying and thinking things that would normally make me cringe or withdraw in disgust is okay. She is unsentimental, but I can tell that she has real compassion for me, so it's possible for me to have some compassion for myself too—and for the child I used to be.

Whenever I ask my family and relatives anything about my childhood, they interrupt me. It was amazing that I *lived,* and it was only because of their vigilant protection of me, and everyone in our family was happy and clever and what's my point anyway, don't I know how hard my mother worked to keep me alive? It all turned out for the best. Just look at me.

"And you were a *happy* child, a really happy child. Always smiling."

One day, on a hunch brought on by a memory I can't figure out—sitting on an examination table, drinking sickly sugar water in front of my concerned-looking mother—I call the hospital and ask for my records. Three weeks later, I receive a pile of pages half an inch thick. These are only the discharge summaries, the pages that have a narrative, not test results and forms. I'm stunned by the sheer volume of pages written about me. They're copies of typewriter carbon copies, some two-sided, signed by a horde of different doctors who met me as a child. The pages detail hospitalizations and my responsiveness to different drugs they apparently tried out, my always-failing weight curve drawn on the printed charts of expected development. I can't believe how tiny I was for years. *Lighter than hand luggage.*

The pages start when I was around six months old. Most are straightforward with hardly a human touch at all.

"Patient is girl of almost four, with hyper allergy to foods, asthma, eczema, suspected cystic fibrosis."

"Mother resistant to cortisone treatment because of side effects."

"They were planning a trip and still want to go."

"Patient is underweight but has strongly developed thigh musculature from figure skating."

I don't seem to have stayed away from the hospital for more than a few months from the time I was a six-month-old baby until I was twelve—and then there's my last hospitalization at fifteen, for asthma, only a few days before finishing ninth grade. My parents took me to the ER on a Friday afternoon and I was out again by late Saturday afternoon. I didn't even miss Monday's gym class. According to my dad, the cortisone injection they gave me meant that my lungs were in better shape than ever for exercise. I remember that night, my first in an adult ward: an old man in the hallway coughed until he retched again and again. I couldn't fall asleep for even a minute, so I kept writing on a pad of paper with a medical logo on it, making the panic worse with every sentence I scribbled about how badly I wanted to go home. Those pages exist somewhere too, probably folded up inside my diary in my mother's attic.

I feel *too* validated, as if I've discovered the nightmares I had were actually real. It would be better if it weren't true and I was just wrong. I want to lie down on the floor under the weight of my medical history and never get up. All these years I've thought of myself as a regular girl with secret stomachaches, shameful exhaustion, coughs, and symptoms, dragging myself around after the other kids to seem normal. But here is overwhelming evidence that I'm not normal, that my childhood was not normal. It's as if there is a whole part of town my family has taken enormous pains to go around, streets and houses that I know so well but have been ignoring and discounting all this time—but it's all right there, waiting to be discovered. *Surely, I can't be expected to be normal considering the abnormality that is my body?*

I bring up the hospital records to my mother one Sunday during dinner in my childhood home. We're seated across the dining room table from each other eating the vegetable soup she has cooked. At first, she seems validated, too—because we're talking about something that was hers and mine, our war stories. About all the work she did. We even laugh a little at first.

But as the conversation goes on, I feel my stomach clench more and more and I eat faster and faster though I know I'll get a stomachache. I try to remember how to talk constructively like I've practiced with Kari, but my body is shutting down. It's as if I'm hoping she won't see me there across the table.

"We just followed the advice we were given," my mother says. "'Act like she's a normal kid. Don't you let her get away with anything,' Doctor Simonsen would say."

"Seriously?" I say. What did I ever get away with?

"You're out to get me too, is that what this is? It's not enough that your father discards me like I'm worthless after thirty years! Don't you dare!"

My mother is still reeling from the separation and these days even the most innocent conversations turn into fights and rants about my father. It appears as if no matter what I do the evenings degenerate in that way. It doesn't even require my participation, though I always say the wrong thing and lose my cool, too. Before long, we're up and running.

"How I labored to make food you could eat! All those meetings we went to! I did the best that I could. God knows your father didn't help. He didn't even believe it was as bad as it was. Thank God for Doctor Simonsen. Don't you remember how we would get up early and take the bus? The *bus*! And walk up that long hill to the hospital because your father *had to have the car*."

I'm crying now and I know I sound angry.

"I didn't even say you did anything wrong! My point isn't that you're horrible or that I blame you. I'm only trying to figure out how to live with this now. I'm clearly not doing it right. I'm not working and still I'm exhausted and every single part of my body hurts."

I can tell from the way her face twists in disgust that she wants no part of this. She wants me to shut up—but I can't.

"I was tiny!" I continue. "You maybe could have occasionally told me, 'We know this is hard for you,' and comforted me. It was dangerous, right? If you 'kept me alive' it means I could have died! It was not *nothing*! You guys pretended it never happened."

"Pretended it never happened?!" My mother throws down her napkin, looking at me in bitter disbelief. "Are you joking? We couldn't eat regular food, any of us! Are you going to complain because we took you on vacation all over Europe? Is that bad too, now?"

I'm still crying. I wipe my nose on my napkin.

She continues, picking up steam: "We tried to give you a normal life! I wanted a normal life, too! Yeah, it's not a fucking secret—we didn't want our lives to be ruled by illness and it's not my fault that it was. It wasn't what we wanted. None of this is what *I* wanted! I couldn't work for years because I was always in the hospital with you! Look at what that's done to my pension rights now that I'm going to have to fend for myself as an old lady. God, I never expected this to happen. To be thrown out of the house like garbage. A letter from a lawyer! 'Vacate the premises!' My own house!"

I begin to noisily stack our plates, cutlery and glasses to clear the table. I'm long since used to her swearing by now, which she never used to do when they were still married. Our whole family feels nuts—nobody is acting like themselves anymore. I could quote that legal letter from memory, that's how many times I've heard this rant. My father's version of what the letter said is different, of course. Their stories never line up.

"Well, I didn't choose to be sick!" I defend myself. "I'm sorry I ruined your life, but you *chose* to have children. I never had any fucking choice in *anything*. And I didn't choose my father. You did! *You* are the one who chose him!"

She looks at me for a moment with a strangely blank look on her face.

"I never would've done any of it had I known," her voice cracks, but she doesn't cry. "I never would've had children. My whole life is wasted." She sits there at the dinner table in the tidy room, wide-eyed and jaw clenched, like she's shocked that what she's said is all true.

"Thanks a fucking million, mom."

The fight goes on as we tidy up, moving angrily around each other in the kitchen, and continues still while my mother brings out the dessert she has prepared—we ridiculously sit down for another meal, as if either of us are going to enjoy it. Apparently, this is normal now. We're both so upset I know it'll take days to recover. While I slam up against the limitations of my value system, my mother is going through something similar—except in her case, she's questioning thirty years of marriage, going through the motions, making sacrifices, acting like a nice lady, and thinking it'll add up and make sense. She assumed that there would be loyalty and a payoff. Her despair and rage could fill her entire suburb.

But I can't fix it for her. I follow Kari's advice two hours too late, telling my mother I have to leave if this fight goes on. She follows me to the door, still ranting about my father until I'm out of the house. She watches me go and slams the door so hard the whole doorjamb shakes. I feel like I can't breathe. I stop in the driveway, out of view of the house, and stand there sobbing for several minutes, wondering whether to go back inside, because I know she would rather keep fighting than be alone. I start walking slowly to catch the bus.

Kari flips through the hospital records for ten long minutes while I squirm on the chair. She places her hand on top of the pages and gives me a look of such warmth and pity that I cringe.

"Medical procedures are horrible and painful for any child," I tell her. "Everyone probably did their best. For any adult, there would be a limit, right? Occasions where the child's agony ranks lower than your own inconvenience and irritation…"

Is it normal to be irritated by agony? I was a very well-behaved child.

"…And all these things were done for my own good, and there were only measured, small cruelties, and only a partial lack of tenderness, kind words, and cuddles to balance and counteract it. There's no way to figure this out, to reach any truth or finish with it, so why harp on about it?"

Kari looks at me and waits. I keep going.

"No one is torturing a kid in the hospital in Norway. It's the minimum amount of suffering in one of the richest countries in the world. It can't be prevented. No point in thinking about it. So those kids just have to fucking tough it out."

"Well, that's what you did, right? You toughed it out."

"Yeah."

Kari looks out of the window for a second before meeting my eyes again.

"But even if it's the minimum amount, it's still suffering, right? It's not outrageous to acknowledge that much. To acknowledge that this was hard on you, *and* on your parents. That as much as it's a story of surviving, of being good and *managing*, it's a story of suffering and sadness, too."

Just as I more or less come to terms with that batch of my hospital records, I pick another equally thick pile out of my mailbox on a sunny afternoon just coming home from town. I drop my backpack and sit down on my lavender duvet and start skimming the pages. For some reason the second stack isn't a chronological continuation of the first one. These pages will need to be shuffled into the first pile.

I read about one more upper endoscopy done in 1984, when I was four. *Which one is it that I remember?* Struggling on the table in a dark room because I was trying to tell them I was choking on the tube and needed to vomit, and instead I was held down by several pairs of hands. The notes only read "uncomplicated access", and further down, "Otherwise, patient is quite active and cheerful." Another two hospitalizations for asthma in 1987. An already unreal feeling I have about these pages is heightened. I can't tell what's what, between the clinical language and the dusky memories I convinced myself I'd made up. I feel like I'm part of some sort of experiment on the nature of memory.

Asthma testing: breathing through tubes with clamps on my nose, holding my breath and then exhaling so hard that I start coughing. Was that spirometry?

Sweat tests: being wrapped in duvets in a small room with my mother next to me, and small electric shocks from the electrodes they attached to my arms afterwards.

Allergy testing: drops of different allergens lined up on the inside of my forearms, a little scalpel-like instrument piercing the skin inside each drop. Watching them swell, grow flecked, bright red with raised, pale welts in the center. Not being allowed to touch them. Feeling them throb all the way to my armpits and that stinging, excruciating itch beyond itching. My mother holding a children's book she brought from the waiting room open over the table where my arms are laid out, trying to keep my interest on it, her voice tense, bright, cheerful. Squirming to sit still and not ruin it so we'd have to start over and do it all again. There was never any way out.

Walking down the smooth linoleum of the children's wing of the hospital to greet a nurse who was old and round and kind. I don't remember her face, but a friendly, deep voice with a Sunnmørsk accent, and her name: Klara. Her gray hair was always up in a bun, her soft arms and a big, round bosom that strained her white uniform. The itchy, icky feeling of smiling politely and handing myself over to them, knowing there was no escape. Undressing to be weighed and measured in my undershirt and underpants. My bare feet on the cold scale and then the clink of the weights being adjusted. Kind voices and smiles letting me know that this occasion was one for smiling, even though there were always needles and adult hands on my body.

I remember the dry skin on Doctor Simonsen's hands most vividly—and his balding head and thick, dark eyebrows and serious eyes, his voice when talking to my mother. It's as clear to me it's as if it's happening right now. I hear her telling me off for not sitting still once when he took a blood sample himself so we wouldn't have to go downstairs to the children's lab and wait in line. He was doing us a favor, but he wasn't good with the needle and it was extra painful, the burning wrongness of that sensation, the sharp metal in my tender skin. I try to hold my breath, it's not like I'm not used to being pricked with needles, not like I'm some *baby*, but I just can't help it, it hurts too much. Tears run down my face as they chat.

My vision goes blurry and I feel hot and nauseous. *Jesus*. I rub my hand against the crook of my arm and shake myself in order to be released from of the pages, back into my sunlit room where I'm an adult who's in control of her body. I'm hot and panicked and I haven't even read through half of the new stack.

Late that evening I watch an episode of The O.C. on my laptop in bed and suddenly find myself crying. It's a stupid show, but I'm actually sobbing and kicking my sheets over how cruelly the poor main character is treated by all those wealthy people around his adopted family. He's different from the rich kids and the way they talk to him, it's as if what they have is deserved—earned—rather than a cruel, random system of which he happened to be born on the outside and they on the inside. *No fucking hope of bridging that gap, just outside forever.* No power over himself. Forever having to put in the extra work and extra explanations, never expecting to be understood. Always on your best behavior, at risk of having even small privileges revoked.

My parents don't know Siri exists. Siri doesn't know anything about my past that's recorded in these two stacks of pages, now hidden in two separate envelopes beneath other papers on my desk.

In good moments, I believe that I can be present for whatever comes, stay in my body, and grow stronger. I want more of that feeling, the feeling that maybe we didn't know what was going to happen after all, that maybe there is beauty where I couldn't see any before—even just in the spotless hardwood floor of my room, where the sun reflects on a clear day. Beauty in clean bedsheets, a tidy kitchen with the evening light coming in, or the low clouds over the city and the seven mountains surrounding it. Or in Nordnes Park, where the trees reach for the sky, so tall, whole, and quiet.

Axel: Considered the toughest jump to triple, because it has an extra half revolution. The skater takes off from the outside edge of the skating foot. The landing is on the back outside edge of the free foot.

There are other parts of my life too. My school friend Marius and I are in Café Opera in the center of Bergen, waiting for Siri to show up. Marius and I were fifteen when we first met, and have stayed close since, even though I haven't seen much of him lately. I'd probably be bothered by this if I wasn't busy with Siri. Marius gets his looks from his gorgeous Ghanaian mother; he stands out in Bergen. He's always been popular. In high school, I had a little thing for him, but was never brave enough to make the first move.

I want them to meet each other before he leaves town. It's the time of the week when people with children take over the cafés—squealing and screaming accompanies the loud music. I'm excited, slightly buzzed from caffeine and last night's hangover. I've been talking eagerly to them both about each other in an attempt to tie different pieces of my life together. I want to show her off to him. I look out the window to see if Siri is coming and glance at my phone to see if she's texted me.

Marius comes back with our drinks. He looks tired. He tries to avoid rattling the cups and saucers on the table, having forgotten spoons and sugar.

Two years ago he dropped out of medical school and then went to business school for a short period. Now, he works as a pharmaceutical rep and travels around using his charms to hand out logo pens and give speeches on drugs. His mode of transportation is a very round company car spray-painted with the logo that I can't help thinking of as a little undignified. While I wasn't looking, he suddenly became a working man, navigating adult territory that I reserve the right to avoid for a few more years. He makes people laugh and want to impress him. Even though I'm no longer fifteen, he has that same effect on me. I suspect he lacks that sliver of self-doubt that would give him any stake in attuning himself to others. Meanwhile, I have too much of that quality, so between us it works. If his looks run out, he might have a problem.

Siri and I met online only last spring, a couple of weeks after I went on sick leave. Miraculously, there she was: the one attractive lesbian roughly within my age group that none of my friends had slept with.

She wasn't even that new to town. The whole thing was so easy: we met in person after only a week of heavy-handed flirtatious messages. She was stunning; half a head taller than me, with short, white-blonde hair that lay smoothly across her forehead, and a handsome, angular face. Her taciturn personality had me talking nonstop. Her sleepy eyes seemed amused and possibly a little sarcastic. We got drunk on red wine in a bar that was all shiny surfaces and quiet conversations; she stood out like a sore thumb with her leather jacket and the chains on her jeans that clanked against the barstool whenever she shifted. It didn't bother me at all that people looked at us when I made her laugh.

I went to the bathroom and greeted my tipsy face in the mirror; my grin showed my bluish teeth and I admired the smoky eyes I'd spent a long time perfecting at home with a tiny amount of glittery white eye shadow in each corner. I could hardly believe that this was my life now—dates with sexy women on clear spring evenings. It fascinated me that you could simply admit to wanting to get laid, that other people had bodies under their clothes all the time. I went back to her room that night. She only had a stereo and a mattress on the floor and the walls were bare, except for a few snapshots of a golden retriever and a fat baby I later learned was her nephew, but everything was very tidy. I leaned close to the photo of the dog, drunkenly and nervously trying to think of something to say, when she grabbed me, put her muscular arms around me, and backed me up against the wall.

Our bodies, so close in size, fit together amazingly well. She has strong, clever fingers, and I can't stop being flattered that she's interested enough to do all those things to me. She has freckled shoulders and tender skin that burns easily when we go swimming. I can't let my guard down with her. She swims up to me under the surface and drags me under, pushes me into the water and then dives in to rescue me, laughing the whole time. When she is turned on, red spots appear on her neck, and her cheeks flush, her narrow eyes taking on a heavy look. Even sitting across from Marius, I'm having vivid flashbacks of the things we did the last time we saw each other. I have bruises blooming in several places.

I pursue sex the same way I do yoga: breathe, focus, and push the boundaries a little. My body feels like it's finally being put to appropriate use and there is no end to my appetites. I'm triumphant. I keep thinking over and over, "*Wow, so this too is something I can enjoy.*"

"Laura, what are you going to do now?" Marius asks.

I pull away from my thoughts and find that I'm smiling.

"What do you mean?"

"This fall, are you going back to the university, or what?"

"I haven't made up my mind yet…They might still have work for me at the tourist information center after the summer."

"What, you're not going to get your degree? Haven't you been gallivanting around for years already?" He smirks, but his voice is serious.

"I will, I just enjoy having a little more time to myself—having time to write, you know? I can always go back to university. I can actually live off what I'm making now. I don't have to rush into things..." I'm *almost* lying, but I don't want to go into so many personal details with him. There'll just be a lot of explanation and judgment if I tell him I'm on sick leave. It would take over the conversation. He impersonates my pre-divorce father rather well, and I'm not in the mood for it. My life isn't so impressive objectively, but I feel pretty good in my own skin.

"I thought you thought literary theory was bullshit anyway," I say.

"I do," he says.

He has the decency to laugh a little.

Siri and I have spent most of the summer in bed or partying. Our relationship is a secret power—shared glances and sniggers with her and my friends, exchanging scandalous stories of what we get up to when we're wasted. We go out dancing at the three gay bars in town, Siri's and my alliance joining different cliques of queers to form a larger entourage than I've ever had. I've been neglecting my parents and forgetting to return phone calls. When I take a day by myself, I mainly catch up on rest. The part of my life that holds everything difficult, complicated and painful can wait. It's as if I've been drunk the whole summer. Even being hungover is fun, because we lounge on her bed and watch illegally downloaded episodes of *The L Word* on her computer all day. Siri finds it hilarious and is delighted with how dirty it is, and I hide how I'm sometimes moved to tears.

It's a new feeling: that *lesbian* is finally something I can do confidently and well. The word used to make me cringe; I could barely say it out loud a few years ago. Now I use it as often as I want and enjoy its effect on people, even though it doesn't describe me perfectly. I find it unlikely that I'll ever date guys again, but I know better than to rule anything out—only a few years ago I was living with Luke. Although women have always been more visible to me than to most girls, it didn't dawn on me that I could actually touch a girl until I was twenty. It's not really a question of whom you sleep with, but of how free you feel. I give anyone who asks the speech about kindly not using their restrictive and artificial labels on me, but for once in my life, I don't care what anyone on the outside thinks of me.

Even as a feminist, I'd never fully realized how much of the derision for women and their bodies had made it into my own mind. It felt deeply radical to just start loving female things. And I could never explain the freedom I felt when I simply stopped trying to be appealing to men and instead tried on some of the things I used to be ashamed of; tasted the sexiness of things that are seen as masculine, weird, embarrassing and ugly, like JD Samson's mustache or Peaches' rude lyrics and hairiness. Abandoning dignified girlness, not just to sleep with women but to dance with no shame, smile without trying to look different, without hiding. Allow something to unfurl slowly and grow from inside instead of trying to snip, shape, and curb myself from the outside. I can use the queer pride language and ideas to allow myself to be all those other things too, things nobody else wants me to be. I can even find strength and a unique perspective there—a sick, queer, nerdy writer. *Stop trying to be normal.* It's like a landslide slowly coming loose—once one thing went, the rest started to slip, whole flakes of the landscape came undone and crashed down with a loud, glorious roar.

Now I'm riding my bike everywhere without makeup on, singing along with my headphones, and feeling strong and happy, like I'm hot stuff. The fact that I can make someone like Siri squirm is delicious. Wherever I go lately I see women and think boldly that I could make them come like a ton of bricks if only they'd let me practice my fabulous skills on them.

"Did you know Marianne knows Siri's ex from school?" Marius asks me.

"Really?" I say.

"Apparently they were pretty serious." He loves sowing discord.

My ears are ringing slightly and the café is noisy. Marius and I were at the same party at my friend's last night, but we didn't talk much there since we were meeting today. I indulged in the triumph of telling the friends I hadn't seen since before summer about Siri. It was so nice to finally have some good news, to laugh at my friends trying to out-crude each other in the kitchen, the two dogs running around our legs. One of them is a shy Vizsla called Stella that I adore. I suddenly remember being asked about Simone de Beauvoir's memoir that I said I would read, but the truth is I haven't touched the book since it was lent to me.

It's drizzling outside now; the café feels moist and there's too little space between the tables. The ends of my pant legs begin to soak through my sneakers and a wave of fatigue and embarrassment about last night catches up with me. *Did I really brag to someone about how frequently and spectacularly I'm getting laid? Did Marius hear me?* My embarrassment transforms into annoyance that Siri hasn't shown up yet.

Just as I try to push away the tired awkwardness at having forced two reluctant strangers to meet, excitement kicks in as I see Siri coming around the corner, walking more slowly than I'd have liked. The sight of her gives me a pleasant jolt. She's wearing the uniform of stylish, young lesbians in our town: jeans worn low, fancy sneakers, and a hoodie under a leather jacket.

A part of me wants to ditch Marius and just go home and fuck her. She enters the café and kisses me straight away. I feel her tongue. She shakes Marius's hand politely and goes to get a coffee. I look at him eagerly, with a too-broad grin, *I can't believe this beautiful creature is all mine.* I want Marius's approval somehow, but when I spot his skeptical gaze and smile of disbelief, I realize he doesn't find her attractive in the least.

I consider Marius. He is wearing all black. His pants look expensive. He has that slumped, pasty look of someone who only experiences his body's existence when hungover. Siri, who works out every other day and openly judges on appearance, won't be impressed by him.

Siri comes back with a coffee cup and sits down. She puts her hand on my thigh under the small table, all of our knees touching briefly. I feel embarrassedly happy, yet hyper-aware of Marius awkwardly looking out of the window as she touches me. I have a suspicion Marius is okay with me being queer, but only if my queerness stays behind closed bedroom doors.

"So, how did you two meet?" he asks, even though all three of us know I have already shared the whole story with him.

Sometimes, I still can't tell when Siri is joking. All her friends are good-looking tough girls like her. A casting director could have assembled them as a photogenic friend group on *The L-Word.* One has short dreadlocks, another a full sleeve of excellent tattoos, and they all have gorgeous lips, graceful necks, white teeth, beautiful breasts, capable hands, strong laughs. I like them so much that the thought that I could have gone with any of them instead of Siri if we'd met under different circumstances has flashed through my mind on multiple occasions.

"So, Laura tells me you're a medical rep?" I hear Siri say as I go to get another coffee for Marius and me.

I can tell they already dislike each other, as they both look up at me with a mix of relief that I'm back and blame for putting them in this situation. Siri stirs and stirs her coffee. The metal on porcelain makes a scraping sound. Silence.

Only twenty minutes later, I've pulled out everything I have to keep the conversation going and my neck and shoulders are stiffening with the effort. Siri and Marius are both shuffling their feet and looking at the table. I recall that I heard Marius mention something last night about what it's like to always be in doctors' offices and decide to throw it in to this conversational stalemate.

"Do you ever wish you'd stayed in medical school?" I ask him.

"No, I'd still be in school, instead of making money. And I'd have to deal with patients. I'm gaining a whole new respect for doctors from seeing the freaks they work with—so many people insisting on sick leave or paid disability for the most ridiculous things. So many people taking advantage of the system. You wouldn't believe the stories."

Siri's interest is piqued.

"Sick leave is on the rise, you know," she says. She's always annoyed with one of her colleagues for taking sick days. She loves to talk about how people should get their acts together.

"It's ridiculous. They really should change the rules. A lot of these people aren't even sick."

I know this whole spiel. I want to cry. There they are, two people in the perfect blossom of their lives, both so invested in their jobs. They could do something else, but it's what they are: *people who work*. I seem to be something else.

One might think their minority status would help them understand, but it's quite the opposite. Siri is gay, yet conventional in every other way. Marius is Black, but he's quick to specify that he's Norwegian—definitely no immigrant or "freeloader". When they look at me, I can tell they don't see any of the things they dislike about "people who take advantage" in me. I'm upset, and they have no idea.

It's a closet moment. I could come clean and simply say, "*I'm* currently on sick leave." They would raise an eyebrow and lose a certain portion of respect for me, and then the polite backtracking would come, of course they don't mean *me! I'm* actually sick, not faking it. This is just a *phase*. I want that to be true, but I also have the urge to rip the Band-Aid off and convince them that I *am* all those things—I *am* sick. Unsexily, chronically so. I want to show them the sheer amount of documents and letters that prove who I am, my current doctor's arguments to the authorities about why my issues are lasting and unfixable so that I'll be granted the extended sick leave. I would change before their eyes into something else, instantly.

None of it is spoken, but I can feel it underneath the surface, the implications of what's occasionally said out loud: *Would you ever date someone who was in a wheelchair? Are you sure you want extended sick leave on your permanent record? You can't need this many breaks. Everyone's tired after work. Being allergic isn't a disability. Period pain isn't an illness. You can't be sick again, you've missed so many days already! These stomachaches must be psychosomatic. Maybe you're just depressed. You should exercise more. Pull yourself together!*

How can those things exist at the same time as the sexy stuff? If only I could be one of those people who only have problems they've seen on TV a million times before, acted out by people who look like them. I could have a script to work with, a way to be stylish about it, different versions to select, not have to invent the shape of the scene from scratch. The only sick people I can remember seeing on TV smile gracefully and then die attractively. They're never angry or bitter, they never feel cheated. They orchestrate beautiful gestures, they head into surgery, content to only say a few well-crafted, self-sacrificing sentences that make everyone else grateful for their own health and then they're gone forever. No abject, terrified misery ever overwhelms them. It's never about the sick person. Whenever anything too unpleasant or painful or—God forbid—to do with the body starts up, the camera cuts away, leaving the sick person completely alone. Never does anyone let on feeling anger so great it can't even begin to be translated into words.

If only I could be what I appear to be sitting here: clean, young, and healthy, right down to each pore of my skin and each strong, flexible yoga muscle down to the bone. No one would suspect me for a second of being ill. "Straight-acting", able to pass. I could at any point prove to some higher authority that I'm *normal*, I'm not one of *those people*. I could hide forever, just clench my teeth and not let on that I'm in pain.

Even though Siri and Marius are finally agreeing on something, I manage to say something.

"How do you know whether those people are faking or actually sick? There could be a lot going on with them that you don't have the faintest idea about."

They both look puzzled.

"Well," Marius sounds annoyed.

"Come on, you have to admit that a lot of people are just lazy assholes," Siri cuts in.

"What?"

"You give people way too much credit." Her tone is harsh. "People will screw you over if you go through life like that."

"Well. *Okay*!" is all I can come up with.

Marius lets out a short bark of laughter at seeing me put in my place by my girlfriend. I'm suddenly sick of both of them. I let the silence linger for a while.

"I have to get going," I say abruptly.

I can feel their gaze on me. I make an effort to keep my face neutral. Siri pulls her leather jacket from the chair. They both follow me outside.

"I'll call you," I tell the space between the two of them before getting on my bike. The drizzle feels good on my hot skin as I ride home.

That evening, the rain pounds the skylight above my mat in the yoga studio, which is quiet but alive with the Ujjayi breathing of twenty people. I'm in a sitting position, bent forward over my legs while my teacher repeats her catch phrase: *"Yoga is about meeting your body wherever it is today."* I use the breathing to ease deeper and deeper into the stretch and feel my body give a little. The stretch, the release in the top-back of my thighs, is made possible by the tautness in the front of my thighs. My belly button draws in toward my spine, fortifying the trunk of my body, enabling me to exert this level of control and release.

In that moment, I feel intensely that this is *my* body, my own personal body—this is, in fact, *me*. Even after I've neglected it for such a long time, it is still there for me. A sob comes from somewhere inside me—a sudden surge of presence, like letting out a breath after being unaware of holding it for a long time—and its release creates more room for me to live in. I continue to push the stretch gently, too much and pain would ruin it immediately. Not too little, either, or nothing would happen. As long as I'm inside the breath and the gentle movement, a little space clears, the landscape flattening so I can see the horizon for a minute.

PART 7

I'M GONNA LOVE YOU LIKE I'M INDESTRUCTIBLE

2003

I'm twenty-two, and I'm living abroad for the first time in my life. My English boyfriend Luke is waiting for me with his French friend, Mathilde, when I arrive in Paris two days after him. He came directly from Reading, where we both live. As I get off the train from London, where I've just been to visit my aunt Elsa, I hear my name—"Laura!"—called out in the distance behind me. Even after six months with Luke, I still love to hear how gentle my name sounds in English. In Norwegian, all the vowels are pronounced separately, the big A and the dip down into U and up again. It exercises the mouth.

Mathilde and Luke are two slim, androgynous people of about the same lofty height, both with short dark hair, dark eyes, and beautiful bone structure. I walk down the platform towards them for ages, too far away to greet them but too close to not acknowledge it. My smile is big. Mathilde keeps hers to herself until Luke makes it clear that I'm the one they're waiting for. He's filled me in on her history with an admiring tone: recurrent cancers since she was sixteen, not to mention openly gay about the same age. I've never known any gay women, and I've never met anyone my own age that has been sick so much, anyone who's been sicker than I have.

I hope Luke remembered to wash his face so I won't have an allergic reaction to kissing him. He cringes when I hug him.

"I've got a toothache," he says.

"What happened?"

There's a slight awkwardness when I extend my hand to Mathilde. She ignores it and puts her cheek against mine and kisses the air next to my face.

"It's been hurting for ages, actually. Probably an inflamed wisdom tooth. I've scored a dentist's appointment in half an hour. Mathilde is going to take you to Roy's place."

Roy is Luke's oldest brother, an actor and the golden boy in their family.

By the look and smell of him, Luke hasn't showered or washed his hair in days. I can't help but feel a little embarrassed in front of Mathilde.

I feel girlish compared to the sleekly self-contained beauties I'm walking with. Mathilde is wearing black cargo pants and a simple dove gray T-shirt that looks elegant on her skinny frame. There's a level of imperfection I can't seem to get, a dirty authenticity that seems to come so easily to other people. Luke has short, spiky black hair, combat boots, and studded leather cuffs that make him stand out back in Reading. He is tall, with broad, sexy shoulders. I want to look tougher, like him. I'm wearing a studded leather bracelet too, that I got from a stall in London. It was so shiny that when I got back to my aunt's apartment,

I made a special trip down to the courtyard to step on it against the gravel to make it look worn and genuine. It still looks brand new, despite all my efforts.

I'm equally drawn to my aunt Elsa's light and tasteful interiors, where everything is clean and made of white linen or smooth wood. For the past two days, I've enjoyed fitting in to my aunt's tidy and well-behaved adult world. I packed my best clothes. Elsa is my only relative outside of Norway—she's my mother's younger sister. I've noticed Elsa is always customizing her clothes, pulling at the sleeves or scrunching them up, popping and straightening collars. Adding a last touch to an outfit with unhurried precision before leaving the house; a necklace, scarf, or a lipstick in a distinct plum or tomato red. She seems to draw an unabashed pleasure from her looks. When I arrived, Elsa touched my hair and frowned for a second before declaring that she loved it. I'd cut it myself into a messy, choppy bob with some purple streaks in it, just before leaving Reading. Beneath my hair, I'm pink-cheeked, my face is smooth and neat like a doll's. No matter what I do, I look innocent, Norwegian, and young. I keep changing my mind as to whether this haircut is perfect or awful.

"Why didn't you go to the dentist before the trip?" I ask Luke. Despite myself, I have my parents in me, always reminding me we can't afford foolishness, vanity, or drama.

"I was going to see my dad's friend for free back home."

We're both always broke and dentists are expensive.

"See you at Roy's later." He turns his handsome face away from me and walks off rather brusquely.

Toe loop: usually the first jump to be mastered, in one of its forms. The skater takes off from the back outside edge of the skating foot, with the help of the toe pick on the free foot. The landing is on the back outside edge of the skating foot. This jump is also called a cherry, or with a small turn (three-turn) just before the jump, a toe walley.

I met Luke while studying abroad in Reading. He's shy, sensitive, and funny, not to mention an entry point into boyish English culture for me. He's introduced me to bacon sandwiches with a thick layer of crisps in them, having the TV on at all hours, taking long baths, and staying in bed all day. Enjoying life, in short. He's in a band and looks sexy playing bass in the local student bars; his striking face, broody demeanor, and excellent outfits make him seem like a real potential rock star. He wears black eyeliner onstage. He's self-deprecating and quick-witted in a way I appreciate but can't contribute to in English. I'm fluent, but half a second slower than natives.

I try to make conversation with Mathilde as we walk towards the apartment where we're going to stay. Her English isn't very good, neither is my French, and the street is noisy, so communication is slow. She has a small, pointed chin and thin, soft hair in a pixie cut that's grown out a little. Her eyes are framed by delicate crow's feet she seems too young to have. She walks with deliberate steps, steadily, with a careful authority. One of her legs is stiff. Despite my good intentions, I keep getting ahead of her as we walk, used as I am to always having to catch up with longer-legged people. It strikes me that I would have had to run to keep up with her too, if I'd met her before her countless surgeries. She looks tough and fragile at the same time. It's as if a small amount of space around her remains unmoved, no one bumps into her like they do me. But she is a puny androgynous girl when it comes down to it, in this city where everyone seems to have a litany of curses at the ready. Immediately, I think I'd kill to prevent an asshole's comment on the street from reaching her. I imagine myself yelling in perfect French for them to shut the fuck up.

But she can take care of herself. I'm the one the guys on the other side of the street shout after. I don't even realize they mean me and I stop, gaping, until Mathilde gently pushes me onward, her touch as light as a wing. I blush and regret my tight jeans, my makeup, anything that makes me a girl. I look out through the bars of the railing down at the Seine, brown in the white light. Mathilde mentions the record-breaking heat wave that we don't know is on its very last day, and its awful results. People have been dying all over the city. I can only manage a shrill cry, "*Mais c'est affreux!*" I wonder if what I said was correct.

Roy's apartment is on the ground floor and is mostly a narrow hallway. There's a small kitchen. It's paid for by the theatre and Roy has the use of the bedroom, which is 75 percent bed. Someone will have to sleep on the floor. Mathilde leaves with a shy smile and a cool wave.

An hour later, Luke stomps into the apartment. From the kitchen table, I hear the bathroom door slam and urine splattering in the toilet.

He comes out and leans on the doorway between the kitchen, hallway and the bedroom. He's pale.

"Hi. How did it go?"

"I have to wait for the antibiotics to work before they can take the tooth out. I'm going to bed," he says.

"You'll probably feel better quickly when the antibiotics kick in."

He's already heading to the bedroom, closing the door.

I stay in the kitchen, reading, trying not to make any noise. Roy comes home later with Mathilde, and they're cooking a simple tomato sauce when I leave the kitchen to go check on Luke. He has discarded his big, dirty army boots right inside the door and now he's in bed on his side, facing the window. There's a sour smell in the room.

"How are you feeling?"

No answer, though I can see that he's awake. I feel a tug of annoyance, but I try to be a good girlfriend and suppress it. People want patience and kindness when they're sick, right? That's what I always wanted. *I'm going to do this better than my parents did.*

"Not so good?"

Still nothing.

"Are you coming out to eat with us?"

"I don't *want* to." Luke's voice is muffled.

I'm unwilling to accept the implications of his statement and after a second, I end up pretending he hasn't said anything.

"Are you feeling terrible?"

He turns over with a look of immense insult.

"I'm *fine*!"

I sit down cautiously on the corner of the bed that is farthest from him.

"You haven't had anything to eat all day, have you? It'll make you feel better. It almost always helps to eat something."

"I'm not hungry."

"You have to eat *some*thing."

"I don't want to eat!"

"I can bring you something if you want."

"Can't you just fucking leave me alone?" He turns over again by kicking ferociously, making the headboard bang against the wall. The low talking and tinkering from the kitchen stops briefly.

I make an effort not to slam the bedroom door and go to the bathroom. I grit my teeth and try not to cry. I'm furious. Even if my arm had been severed, I would have never gotten away with that kind of behavior. My mother would've told me to kindly get a *hold* of myself.

Later, I step out to a smelly phone booth to call my aunt Elsa.

"Luke is being really pissy about his tooth," I can't help blurting out.

"You know, you're more of a pro at being sick than most people your age. He might not have any experience with this kind of thing. Being sick is hard. You'd know, right?"

This defense strikes me as profoundly unfair to me. I'm giving him much better stuff than I ever got. It's as if no matter what, I lose.

I've told Luke about being sick as a child and how badly I wanted someone to see me. To be *not alone*, not the sole owner of all my trouble. But I haven't thought of myself as a sick person in a while.

I've been healthy ever since I left Norway six months ago, the worst has been period pain. Granted, I often let my stomach go past hungry to cramping when I'm out somewhere because I don't want to eat my eternal pre-packed sandwiches in front of people. I know it's not good, because I'm much too skinny, but I don't take any chances when eating. I'm deadly afraid of an allergic reaction alone or around strangers. I just have to make sure it doesn't happen.

I don't think Luke thinks of me as a sick person. Obviously, my allergies require a level of kitchen precision that doesn't come naturally to him. Also, he has to wash increasingly carefully before kissing me. Now even a hug before he's washed can give me a swollen, painful rash on my cheek. *Is it just going to keep getting worse?* I bat away these kinds of thoughts. Sometimes he gets cranky from too many adjustments. I hate needing this from him so much that it makes me angry to even hear him refer to it, not to mention the debt of gratitude he thinks I owe him. I can't get around needing special treatment, no matter what I do. Best not to think of any of this any more than absolutely necessary.

"But, you know," my aunt says, "in life, it's important to choose a partner that brings out the best in you."

I hear her raised eyebrow.

Luke finally feels a bit better and we head to the music festival with Mathilde, as planned. PJ Harvey is onstage. She's wearing a silver dress, and she looks tiny and tough. The music vibrates through my body.

At the end of the night, Mathilde offers to help carry my stuff and asks if I'm tired. She pronounces my name carefully. I am exhausted and have had a stomachache for hours, but it wouldn't have occurred to me to say anything. When I nod, she gives me a small smile like she sees it and knows how I feel.

I feel weird. She is some entirely new kind of fascinating to me. As soon as we get to her apartment, Luke and I collapse on the kitchen chairs. Mathilde puts on some loud Japanese punk music and gets out a dried sausage, bread and vinaigrette to eat with leftover tuna salad from earlier. The fluorescent light in the kitchen is so bright it hurts.

She gets up suddenly to stop the CD, which has started skipping in the other room. Her movements seem painful but are surprisingly elegant. Her bad leg is extra stiff after a long day on our feet and she drags it against the floor before gaining control of it. I can tell none of this is new to her. She fastens her eyes somewhere past the door and keeps them there for as long as it takes to be free of the table and make it out of the kitchen. Her face is tense and blank in the white light. *Does she feel embarrassed, when we jump up to move things out of the way for her?*

The thought makes me want to cry. I want her to transcend my own limitations. I want her world to be full of clear vivid colors, easy trust, and people she isn't afraid to put in their place, should they step on her boundaries. She has earned her citizenship to that place. I don't want her story to be that one where she, after describing the pain in detail, can't think of a thing to say about the good years. Not a thing except to list the classes she took at university, and the names of the people she met.

It's time for Luke and I to go see Roy's play, the main reason we're in Paris. Luke is still quiet, but he looks much better. I make a mental list of compliments I can use even if the play is terrible, but Roy is magnificent. His handsome face looks even better in makeup under the bright stage lights. Afterwards, Luke and I go around to the stage exit inside the courtyard.

"It was good, right?" Luke says in a tense voice.

"It was great!"

"Should we go into his dressing room?"

"Do you think we should?"

"I'll have a fag first. He's really a star, isn't he?"

"Yeah, he wiped the floor with those other guys."

"Yeah."

"He was in a different league."

"Mm."

"We'll just wait."

"Yeah."

We wait, leaning against the wall beside the door. By the time Roy appears (with drawn-on eyebrows and stage makeup) to graciously accept our praise, I've lost touch with the magic of the performance and the words feel empty in my mouth.

We end up in a bar with some of Mathilde's friends and she leans over the table, so I can hear what she says over the music and noise. Her soft cheek brushes against mine as she speaks directly into my ear in English, to make sure I understand. Her heavily accented English is so angular, the bar so noisy, I can barely grasp it in the loud room. She's telling me about her ex-girlfriend, who writes poems about death. She leans back and gives me such a meaningful look that if it were anyone else I would've recoiled. But she knows what she's talking about. *Give us a smile. Just one more.*

Years of rain, then a dry afternoon, to rest on the balcony in the waning sunshine, look out over the landscape, leaves falling from the trees. People want you to believe everything has meaning, that everything is for the best, but it's not true, it's not true at all.

Mathilde is leaving for Nancy in the afternoon, to visit her parents. After strolling around the flea market in Porte de Clignancourt for over an hour, she and I sit down in a café while Luke rifles through records in a booth across the street. She and I haven't talked much. Luke is almost back to his normal self, making us laugh. Mathilde lights up like an entirely different person when she laughs; her eyes become happy slits and dimples appear in her cheeks. I want to make her laugh. She runs her slim hand through her hair and leans against the wall behind her for a few seconds with her eyes closed.

I watch her unabashedly. I imagine myself kissing her eyelids more gently than I've ever done anything. I imagine running my hand down slowly, from her silky hair to her neck, down under the collar of her faded, military green T-shirt. She opens her eyes, and I lower mine. She orders a coffee, smiles, takes a deep breath and asks me what I like to do for fun.

I need to talk to her now that I have her all to myself. I am on the verge of confessing it; the words are already standing in the hallway with shoes and coat on, ready to leave my mouth once and for all. I shift in my seat and sip my Perrier, fumbling for what to say. She looks at me with a kind expression. Then we both look out at the street where Luke is crossing towards us.

We accompany her to the metro station. On the way, Mathilde giggles. It's the least likely sound for her to make in the entire world. "Barbie is a slut," she says in her pointed French accent. It's printed on a T-shirt at a booth. She's earned all the silly behavior she can ever spend. We smile at her.

Luke and I are both tired and hungry by the time we head back alone at dusk. I feel stiff and brittle; any disturbance can turn dangerous. We've scarcely spoken for the past hour. We take a wrong turn and end up in a dark crooked alley far below the bridge we should be crossing. It looks like the kind of street where Shakespearean characters were murdered. We start to turn back, and the prospect of having to walk up the long hill again—on top of the rest of the way home—is grim. We both have painful blisters. I stare crankily at the world as we start climbing the hill again, and that's when a middle-aged man in a suit bumps into me and doesn't apologize. When I turn to look, he gives me a rude, disapproving look over his shoulder. He clearly thinks I'm a disgrace for some posh, French reason.

He's quickly lost in the crowd again.

I'm suddenly beside myself with anger. "What the *fuck* was that," I spit out at Luke, voice furious and thighs aching from the steep climb on the cobblestones in the dark alley.

"What happened?"

"That man slammed into me!"

"He's just a wanker. The world is full of them."

"You know what, fuck this fucking city."

"Pretty much everyone thinks this is the best city in the world," Luke says, stupidly.

I feel a pang of hunger as we climb the last of the hill. "What a *fuck*ing *bast*ard!"

"Can't you ever just let anything go?" Now Luke is pissed off. He doesn't look at me. I drop his hand angrily, my face a tense knot. We push through the never-ending crowd, feeling exhausted, my stomach complaining along.

I take his hand again, because it's easier to move through the throng together. I scan the crowd irritably and notice a handsome, sickly-looking man in his thirties moving towards us slower than the rest. His blazer is loose like he's recently lost weight and he has an earring in one ear. He looks a little familiar. I think of the protesters during the AIDS crisis of the '80s. Those emaciated, androgynous men on TV always moved me; loudly and angrily fighting for their rights as frail sick people, right there in our living room, where I laid on my stomach on the floor close to the TV, looking and looking at their fiery eyes, while my parents huffed disapprovingly from the sofa behind me.

Those men had friends, lovers, brave sidekicks standing next to them. Antonio Banderas in *Philadelphia* pops into my head; handsome, warm-eyed, the empathy so vivid on his face, rushing to the hospital to defend Tom Hanks against the doctor who wants to put him through an unnecessary colonoscopy, the first time I'd ever heard that horrible word said on TV. *You need someone to be out there in the cold, dark night alongside you.* All the fragile, sick, gay people out there in the world living their lives, even though many people don't like them. Going through their days, kissing and tenderly touching and working and making art and owning moments that are only theirs. *Something in me feels so sore.*

As we pass, the man looks at Luke with a gaze of such lonely, eloquent longing it makes my stomach ache. I feel myself shrink next to the version of Luke the man sees. Luke's long lashcs and big hands, veins popping on his forearms; his potential for advanced and adult sexual things I can't even imagine. He also looks like a strong and tender champion for a sick person to lean on, like he could help and love and take care of you and never run out of energy and compassion. He looks like exactly what you'd want. Maybe he could be. Maybe for someone else.

The next morning, it's still the two of us, going back to our lives together in England. The train station is in complete chaos because of a strike. Our train back to London is delayed, and for some reason it's stalled at the beginning of the platform. Hundreds of stranded, angry passengers run toward the train as fast as they can, struggling with their luggage. Luke and I can't get close enough to find out what's going on. We're too tired to even try. We go inside the station to sit down and wait however long it'll take before another one comes along.

PART 8

DO SOMETHING PRETTY WHILE YOU CAN

1995

It rains for 244 days of the year in Bergen because of the seven mountains that surround the city and catch every rain cloud from the North Sea. If you ever see a picture of the city, you won't be able to tell, because everyone who lives here only takes photos when it's sunny. When the sun comes out, everyone rushes outside, immediately. Ladies stand on street corners, turning their faces to the light like flowers. The entire figure skating season, except for a few days in the beginning of October, is dark, cold and wet. But you would never know, if you flicked through my parents' photo albums.

I'm walking home from school alone when Linda, who shares rides to figure skating with me, catches up. The lenses of my glasses are wet because, of course, it's raining. I glance over my shoulder to make sure no one from my class sees me talking to a twelve-year-old, but I'm already pretty far from school, so there's no one around. *Still, it's so annoying.*

Linda is my only friend at figure skating, and although I'm fourteen, I look just as young as her, because I'm so short and skinny.

Linda talks openly about anything like words are of no consequence. Like it takes hundreds of them of them to communicate anything.

"Can't they drink milk in your classroom?"

"No," I explain, though I know Linda already knows what the deal is. The school sent a letter to all the parents in my class about the milk room, informing everyone of what a freak I am. "The other kids in my class have to drink milk in a different room because I'm super allergic. If I get even a drop of it on my skin, a blister breaks out right away and it hurts like hell."

When it happens , it feels like the skin is about to split open, the kind of pain that demands that you deal with it immediately. Even if I run and wash it off, the bright red swollen rash stays and keeps hurting and itching, the whole limb throbbing. When my family travels, we carry a plastic emergency kit that looks like a red lunchbox, but it has needles and little glass bottles of adrenaline and cortisone in it.

My mother thinks I don't want people to feel sorry for me, but I do. I can't remember ever wishing there was less pity. There's a small carton of milk for each kid. They put the milk in a small room off of our classroom and all the kids go there to eat their lunches and drink it. This means I'm usually left alone in the classroom to eat my packed lunch. Sometimes I trail into the doorway of the milk room until someone tells me I shouldn't be there.

"Torbjørn said it couldn't possibly be that bad. That you're spoiled. Like, why does your mother make such a big deal? He said she sounds like she has a screw loose." Linda is sort of pretending to take my side by telling me what he said. She is always realigning her loyalties and she's not subtle. Her foster dad, Torbjørn, has such a friendly, tired face that it's horrible to think of him saying that about me and my mother. The worst crime in my house is making a big deal of yourself. Not just in my house, in my school, too. Everywhere.

We are walking up a hill, with houses on both sides. The rain makes a tiny river that creates fan shapes down the tarmac like a little staircase under my feet. I kick the gravel and water with every step. I start cursing. "My mother is not crazy! How dare he. What an asshole. What an ASS–HOLE! It's dangerous for me, why doesn't he get it? I could DIE! I'm *that* allergic! I could die, and people won't even understand it!"

Linda looks at me, mystified and wide-eyed, like I'm performing some unknown ritual. I can't make her understand. *She's so dumb.* My tantrum is long over by the time our paths diverge, though I stretch it out and keep kicking the ground for as long as I can stand to.

When I get home, my mother is making dinner with the local radio news playing loudly, to be audible over the frying pan and kitchen fan. She greets me distractedly. She is turning Pollock fillets over in a plate of my bread mix with salt and pepper and then frying them. The already golden fillets in the frying pan are surrounded by rings of sweet, yellow onion. Potatoes are boiling on the other burner. I hug her from behind and lean my face against her white knit sweater between her shoulder blades, breathing in the scent of her perfume and skin. My mother is surprised and turns halfway towards me with a pleased smile that turns a little worried.

"Hei!"

She pets my hair with her wrist, since her left hand has fish and flour on it and her right hand holds the spatula. Her eyes search my face for a second. Satisfied that I'm okay, she asks me to grate the carrots for dinner.

We're in the dressing room at the ice rink, a long, narrow room with wooden benches on both sides, waiting for the ice to be prepped. The hockey boys are overtime, slamming into the boards and yelling, leaving bloodstains on the ice, cutting into the figure skaters' rink time and making everyone antsy. Then they rumble down the hallway, banging things and shouting like they're twice as big and twice as many as they really are. The other girls smooth their ponytails and tightly lace and re-lace their skates while they wait.

On Mondays and Wednesdays, our coach is Nina. She's sixteen and has plucked her eyebrows into half-circles that are uniformly millimeter-thin all the way. She wears lots of black eyeliner and her thick hair is bleached yellow. She is like a doll. Her perfect figure skating body underneath her mean face is clad in a tight leotard and big, cut-off gym pants made of crackly synthetic material on top. She wears leg warmers on her skates, like Tonya Harding wore off the ice at the Lillehammer Olympics last year. She is only one year older than me—but in this situation I am lumped in with the younger girls. I'm glad not to be judged by her standard and keep my mouth shut most of the time.

Nina is kind of nice to us in practice, but always makes it clear that she doesn't like us, like an unhappy mother yelling at her kids on the bus. Today she's pissed because she can't go train with a visiting coach from Russia along with the other older girls because she has to train us. We're huddled on the benches in our exercise clothes, while Nina complains to her friend Silje, who sometimes helps her out with the coaching and provides disgusted facial expressions and scornful laughter. I'm reading a book and trying to hide it in the tent of my hanging jacket like I just happen to be searching for something in the depths of it. Luckily *The Babysitters' Club* books are small so it's half-possible. I read in English because I have a good ear for language, everyone says. I only tune in when I hear words that make me hot with shame.

"...with these brats who don't even have their periods yet!"

And Linda, who never knows when to lay low, says: "I have! I'm having my period right now."

"Ha! So that's why it smells like dog in here!" Nina laughs and Silje joins in.

Linda's face falls. Why doesn't she get it? You can't win. You never mention your period—or, if you do, you do it with a show of shame. Extra shame can't hurt. Better that than thinking you're something you're not, someone whose body can do something that isn't disgusting. I slide my book into my bag and leave the dressing room, praying they won't comment. I go to lean on the boards and watch the Zamboni slowly lick the surface with warm chemicals to give us silky smooth new ice.

A lack of courage to go big and really jump is the main hindrance to getting better, according to Aleksey, our main coach. He is Russian. We can all get ourselves high up off the ice with our strong legs, but landing elegantly or even safely is worse. It's nuts. The deep grooves the hockey players leave can't be erased in that one round of the Zamboni between their time and ours, and sometimes they turn our forceful and elegant jumps into spectacular falls. Your skate sticks in a groove and suddenly all your power conspires to crack your chin or elbows against the ice.

You have to go so high to get the whirl that there is no safe way to do it. You have to give everything you have and risk your tailbone and complete humiliation to execute a beautiful jump.

My unspoken burning desire is just to be able to do something beautiful using my body. I fantasize about having control of the music and the ice rink to myself. The ice rink is like a cathedral: that high ceiling, the way the sound echoes in the chilly, clean air. My body is a hard twig of muscle, with the pronounced thighs and buttocks all figure skaters develop, and tiny, secret breasts. My pride is my hair, which is an unglamorous ash blonde color, but very long, smooth, and shiny. *I can't wait to get contact lenses and learn to wear makeup and become the closest thing to pretty that I possibly can.* My mother bought me a pin from the Lillehammer Olympics, a figure skater portrayed in the cave painting style they used for all the Olympic stuff.

I manage to grab the unusual privilege of being first and alone out on the ice for a few minutes. I start on the warm-up rounds, loving the speed. I switch effortlessly from the inside edge to the outside and turn. I am contained inside my movement. The small space I occupy; my firm thirty-six kilos of muscle and sinew work flawlessly. For every single movement, my strong thighs shift me forward, spectacularly fast and far. Chest and head up, smile on my face, hands out parallel with the ice. I own the entire ice rink and take up all that space, feeling the cool air on my cheeks and my tight ponytail fly out behind me.

I swivel backwards with a soft crunch of the pick of my skate, into my favorite position: gracefully speeding backwards, but turning my head to face forwards haughtily, like a flamenco dancer, my arms positioned forward and backward along the clean line of the movement, against the flow of cold air. I adjust my head so my hair is out of my face, but a few silky strands always tickle my cheeks. Then I straighten up and swiftly round the short end while moving forwards; I take on the long side again and have one round done already. *I could do this forever.*

The others catch up and start their warm-up around me, filling the enormous space with the crisp, clean incisions of steel skates on fresh, white ice.

I love to push against the limits of my body. It's small and unremarkable, but it can do things. We stand against the railing high above the rink on the second floor, doing ballet exercises. *Stand on one leg, hold the rail next to it, the other arm up. Tighten your core, shoulders back and chest up, face up, always with a composed expression. Bend the knee of the foot you're standing on, squat as low as possible and stretch the other foot straight out in front of you, without slumping or touching the floor. Then, remaining in control, swing back up and point that foot up and out behind you in a "flyer".* It's easier with out the weight of the skates on our feet. We're used to the burn in our thighs. I like feeling the burn, and how much easier this is than it used to be last year.

There's nothing I can't do if I put my mind to it and put the time in. Even though my current situation is on the sucky side, the world is malleable, I'm still growing. I'm quite sure I'll get prettier. Within a few years, we all will settle into the heavier bodies of our mothers and sisters. But for now, we're inventing our own bodies, graceful and slender and strong, and we have long hair and porcelain skin and red lips. We can do whatever we want.

I have earned some good times to come. We stand there swinging up and down, trying to look up and ahead, and dream of how good it's going to be.

ACKNOWLEDGEMENTS

My sincere gratitude:

To the many doctors, nurses and other health care workers who have helped me over the years, and to all doctors, nurses, researchers, health care workers and activists who work daily to fight back the wall of human suffering one centimeter at a time.

To my brilliant agent Maria Cardona, Anna Soler-Pont and everyone at Pontas Agency.

To my sharp-eyed and patient editors: Jennifer Baumgardner, Nathan Connolly, Amelia Collingwood, Marte Finess Tretvoll and John Erik Riley, for believing in this book.

To everyone at Cappelen Damm, Dead Ink Books and Dottir Press.

To Taryn Mann for the beautiful illustrations.

To Joanna Hershon for the idea for the structure and for all your help and encouragement.

To Paul Beatty for your teaching and for your support at that crucial moment.

To Donald Antrim, Gary Shteyngart, Øyvind Pharo, Øyvind Rimbereid, Tormod Haugland, Tone Hødnebø, Svein Jarvoll, Joanne Ahola, Isis Medina, Betty Nelly Szlachter, Olav Kise, Heidi Ann Fiske, Giuseppe Daverio, Elise Langsam, Martin Marsteen Williams, Anton Langebrekke, Synnøve Sætre-Hanssen and Kåre A. Hanssen.

To my supportive friends, especially Camilla Bogetun Johansen, Alexandra Kleeman, Lauren Wilkinson, Suchi Rudra, Elin Rødseth, Solveig Askvik, Hilde Taule, Eliza Schrader, Ida Jackson, Hilde Ousland Vandeskog, Martine Dahle Huse, Tonje Li, Rebecca Hinde, George Costigan, Ilka Pinheiro, Ingeborg Sætre-Jørpeland, Margrete Sætre Hanssen, Lauren Schenkman,

Tatiana Gutheil (for letting me steal your beautiful name even though this isn't you), Zoë Harris, Sari Cunningham and the rest of the OWLs.

To Julia Grønnevet and Eirik Forus for helping me get in to Columbia and survive the early days in NYC, and to Rachel Morgenstern-Clarren, Shai Davidai, and other NYC friends who helped me move out of 13K when I couldn't come do it myself.

To my amazingly talented writing group for reading this book so many times: Kevin Magruder, Tom Gottlieb, Scott Dievendorf, and Joe Ponce. To Hala Alyan, Madeline Stevens and Iris Martin Cohen, who also kindly answered my desperate texts and emails on so many occasions, and especially to Yardenne Greenspan for your generosity, sense of humor and all round top notch friendship.

To C.Y. Frostholm, Jan Grue and Mari Wold Sannerud (a gift and a treasure), for your friendship and for providing invaluable encouragement just as I needed it the most.

To my family:

To Gro, for your help with many translation emergencies, for being so sharp and funny and for being a kindhearted big sister especially when I was tiny. To Heidi for being a rock and for getting it.

To my father, who is always ready to listen and who has always been there for me.

And to my mother, who has fought for me tooth and nail ever since I was born, even at great cost.

Last but not least, to Andreas Sætre Hanssen, for the millions of ways in which you made writing this book possible and for all the good and all the bad times.

About Dead Ink

Dead Ink is an innovative independent publisher dedicated to bringing readers bold new books from the best emerging literary talent. Supported by Arts Council England, we're focussed on developing the careers of new authors.

Our readers form an integral part of our team. You don't simply buy a Dead Ink book, you invest in the authors and the books you love. You can keep up to date with the latest Dead Ink events, workshops, releases and calls for submissions by signing up to our mailing list.

deadinkbooks.com

@deadinkbooks